SHADI OWEDA

# Reversing Type 2 Diabetes- My True Journey to Health and Transformation

*A Step-by-Step Guide to Reclaiming Your Health, Achieving Lasting Weight Loss, and Building a Fulfilling Life*

# Contents

# Prologue

In this book, I share the story of how I took control of my health, reversed my Type 2 diabetes, lost weight, and regained the freedom I thought I had lost forever. It wasn't easy, and it didn't happen overnight, but with determination, self-research, and a commitment to change, I found a path to healing that didn't rely on medications or temporary fixes. Instead, I embraced a lifestyle shift that transformed my body, my mind, and my life. I'm here to tell you that reversing Type 2 diabetes is not just a dream – it is possible. You don't have to settle for a life of dependency on medication or face the daunting future that the condition promises.

This book is my blueprint, and I'm sharing it with you so that you too can take back control of your health and live a life of vitality and freedom. In the pages that follow, you will learn the exact steps I took – from crafting a personalized diet plan, incorporating intermittent fasting, and embracing regular exercise, to staying motivated during setbacks and adopting a mindset of success. You'll discover how small changes, when done consistently, can lead to life-changing results. If you've ever felt overwhelmed, defeated, or unsure of where to start, this book will guide you through every stage of your journey. It's time to take action, transform your health, and reclaim your life.

I'm living proof that you can do it – and I'm here to help you every step of the way. So, if you're ready to make a change and take control of your health once and for all, let's dive in.

# Introduction

**My True Journey to Health and Purpose**

**Why I Wrote This Book**

Have you ever felt trapped in your own body, burdened by constant fatigue, aching joints, and the overwhelming fear of an uncertain future? I know exactly how that feels.

Not too long ago, I was living in a cycle of poor health, unbalanced blood sugar levels, and a body that seemed to betray me every day. Type 2 diabetes had taken hold of my life, and my doctor's prescription for lifelong medication felt like a never-ending sentence. But I refused to accept this as my reality. I refused to give up.

In this book, I share the story of how I took control of my health, reversed my Type 2 diabetes, lost weight, and regained the freedom I thought I had lost forever. It wasn't easy, and it didn't happen overnight, but with determination, self-research, and a commitment to change, I found a path to healing that didn't rely on medications or temporary fixes. Instead, I embraced a lifestyle shift that transformed my body, my mind, and my life.

I'm here to tell you that reversing Type 2 diabetes is not just a dream – it is possible. You don't have to settle for a life of dependency on medication or face the daunting future that the condition promises.

This book is my blueprint, and I'm sharing it with you so that you too can take back control of your health and live a life of vitality and freedom.

In the pages that follow, you will learn the exact steps I took – from crafting a personalized diet plan, incorporating intermittent fasting, and embracing regular exercise, to staying motivated during setbacks and adopting a mindset of success. You'll discover how small changes, when done consistently, can lead to life-changing results.

If you've ever felt overwhelmed, defeated, or unsure of where to start, this book will guide you through every stage of your journey. It's time to take action, transform your health, and reclaim your life.

I'm living proof that you can do it – and I'm here to help you every step of the way. So, if you're ready to make a change and take control of your health once and for all, let's dive in.

1

# Chapter 1: The Beginning of My Struggle

## Feeling Off and Unwell

It began subtly, like a quiet voice in the background. I started noticing physical changes in my body—things I could no longer brush off as just tiredness or a rough day. The fatigue was unlike anything I had experienced before, a heavy, unshakable exhaustion that lingered no matter how much I rested. My muscles ached, my joints felt stiff, and my energy levels plummeted.

I was sleeping excessively, hoping that rest would bring some relief, yet I never woke up feeling rested or energized. The constant lethargy weighed on me, making it hard to stay motivated at work or even engage in basic daily activities. What was once a vibrant routine turned into a constant struggle to get through the day.

But it wasn't just the fatigue. I started noticing other troubling signs; frequent urination disrupted my nights, leaving me even more drained during the day. This, combined with an overwhelming sluggishness, only heightened my frustration. My general health was declining, and it was starting to take a toll not just on my body but also on my mental well-being.

## Symptoms That Raised Concern

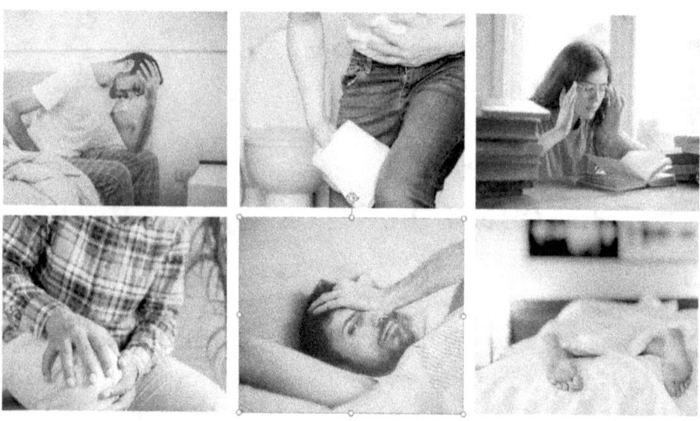

- Increased fatigue and sluggishness, making even small tasks feel monumental
- Persistent muscle and joint aches that limited my mobility
- Frequent urination that disturbed my sleep and drained my energy.
- A lack of motivation to perform well at work or engage in social and personal activities
- A general decline in both physical and mental health that I could no longer ignore.

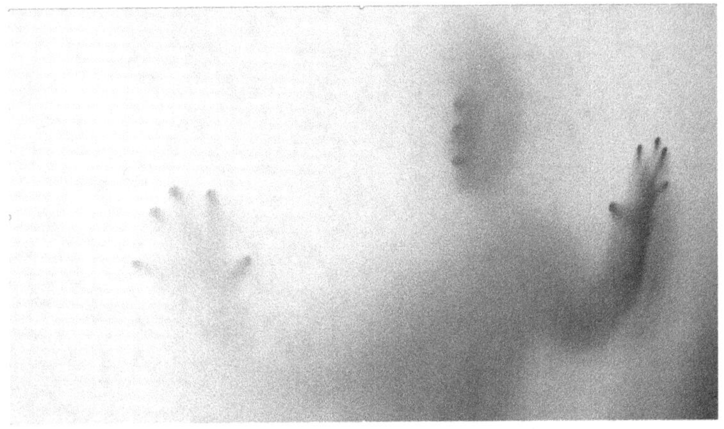

## The Wake-Up Call

The turning point came when these symptoms became impossible to dismiss. I was frustrated and confused, trying to understand why my body was behaving this way. Every day felt like a losing battle against an invisible force that kept me from living the life I once enjoyed

Eventually, I hit a moment of realization. The signs were clear; something was deeply wrong with my health, and it was up to me to take control.

Ignoring the problem wasn't an option anymore. This was my wake-up call, the moment when I decided that I needed to act and regain control over my life.

# 2

# Chapter 2: The diagnosis – A Turning Point

## The Doctor's Visit and Diagnosis

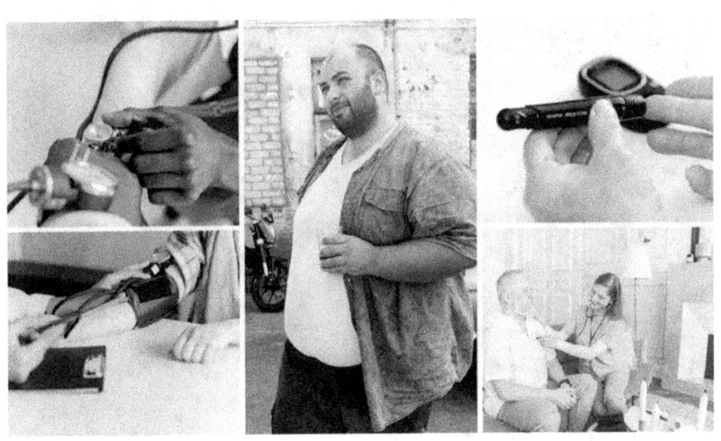

I t was during a routine check-up when everything changed. The doctor sat me down and, after reviewing my test results, faced me with the harsh reality.

I was overweight, my blood pressure was high, and my cholesterol levels were concerning. But the most alarming part came when the doctor measured my blood glucose level. It was 13 mmol/L; far above the normal range.

I remember the feeling of numbness when he said the words, "You have Type 2 diabetes." I had heard about diabetes before, but hearing it applied to me was something entirely different. The doctor handed me a gadget to measure my blood sugar levels daily and explained that I would need to monitor my condition closely from then on.

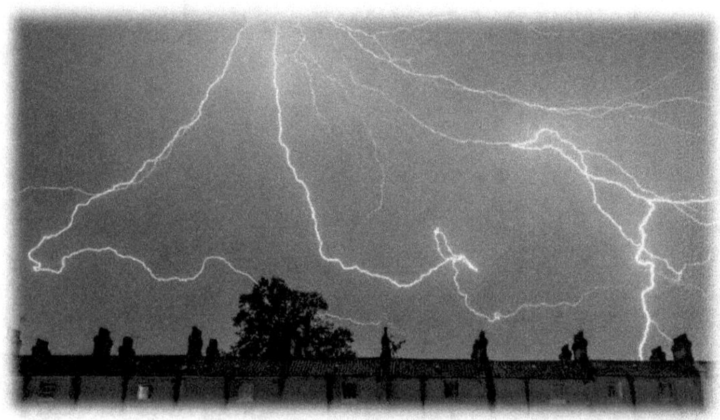

## The Moment of Shock

As the diagnosis sunk in, I was flooded with emotions-shock, confusion, and even denial. I felt overwhelmed, not only by the news itself but by the realization that I would need to make drastic changes in my lifestyle. The weight of the diagnosis began to settle in: this was no longer a matter of just managing my health; it was a lifelong challenge.

Part of me felt relief, though, in having an explanation for how I had been feeling. The fatigue, the unexplained weight gain, the constant aches and pains; it all suddenly made sense. But the relief was short-lived. The thought of living with this condition forever, with the complications that could come later, was terrifying.

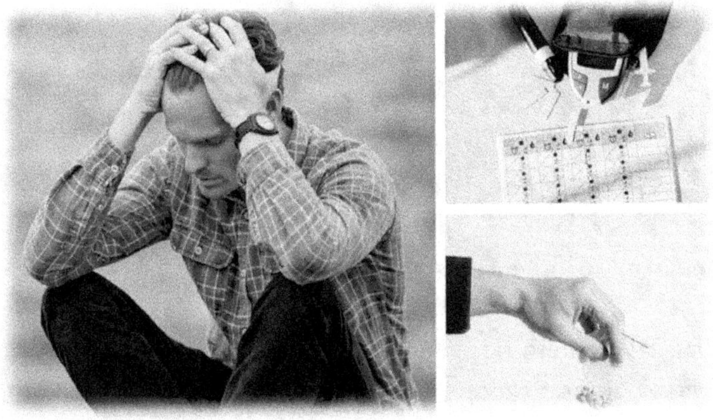

## The Doctor's Plan

The doctor's plan was clear: lifelong medication to manage my blood sugar levels and other related health issues. He spoke of medications I would need to take every day for the rest of my life, a reality I wasn't prepared for. To hear that my body had reached a point where I would need medications indefinitely was both humbling and unsettling.

I felt a mix of frustration and helplessness. How did I get here? But more importantly, was there another way? Could I reverse this condition without relying on lifelong medication? These were the questions that started to swirl in my mind.

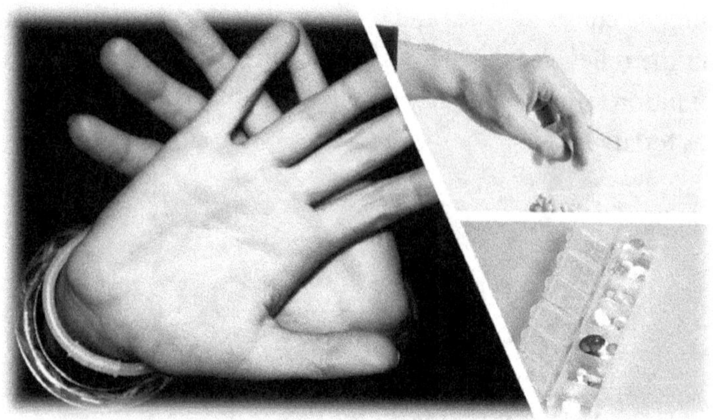

## Deciding to Take Action

That day, something changed within me. I made a decision— I wasn't going to accept this diagnosis lying down. I refused to let diabetes define my future. I wasn't ready to accept the medication route without exploring all my options.

I began thinking about how I could take control of my health, how I could start making the changes necessary to reverse this condition.

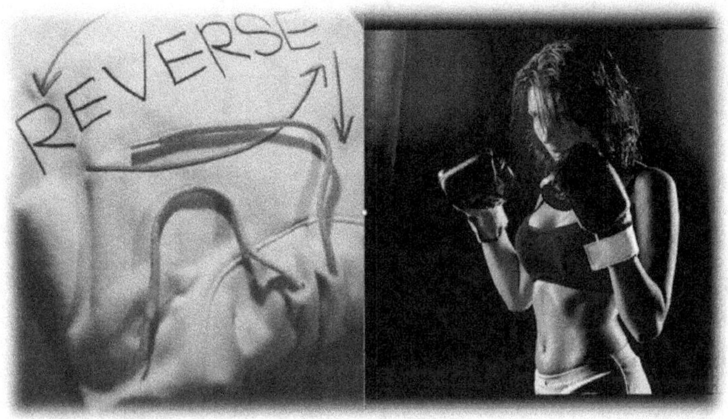


It was time to take action, to fight for my health, and to see if it was possible to reverse Type 2 diabetes through lifestyle changes. I had a long journey ahead, but I was determined to start it that very day.

3

# Chapter 3: Taking Control

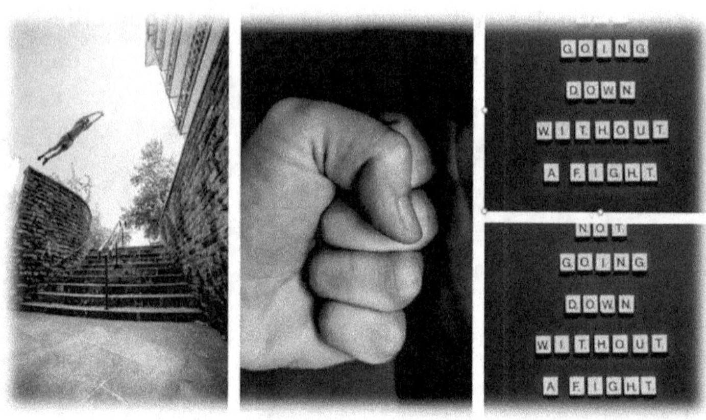


## My Decision to Refuse Medication

When the doctors told me I would need medication for life to manage my Type 2 diabetes, I felt an overwhelming sense of anger. The idea of being dependent on medication forever was not something I was willing to accept.

I made a decision that day I would take control of my health and change my life.

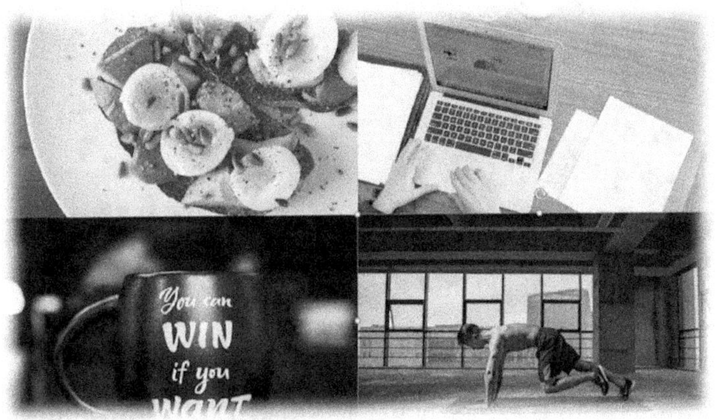


## Turning Anger into Motivation

Instead of letting my anger defeat me, I decided to use it as motivation. I began researching everything I could about Type 2 diabetes, nutrition, and lifestyle changes. I knew I had to act, and I couldn't wait for the doctor's prescription to dictate my future.

So, I developed my own plan, beginning with changes to my diet, exercise, and daily habits.

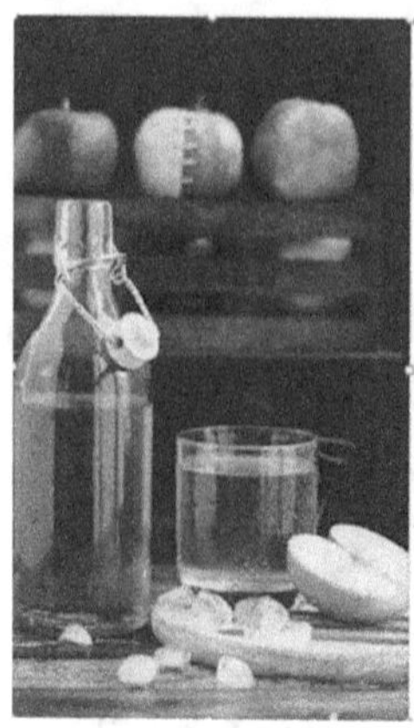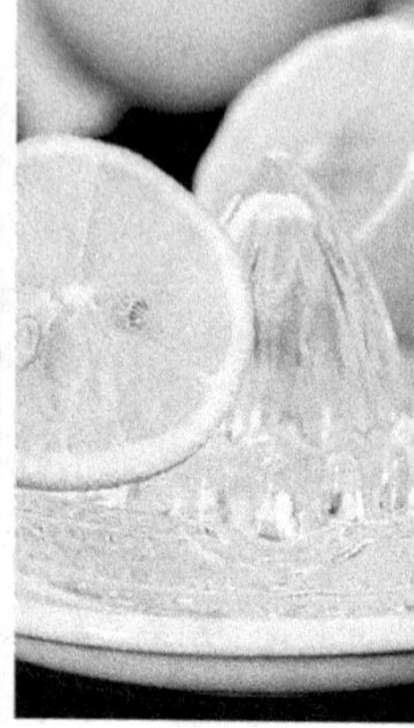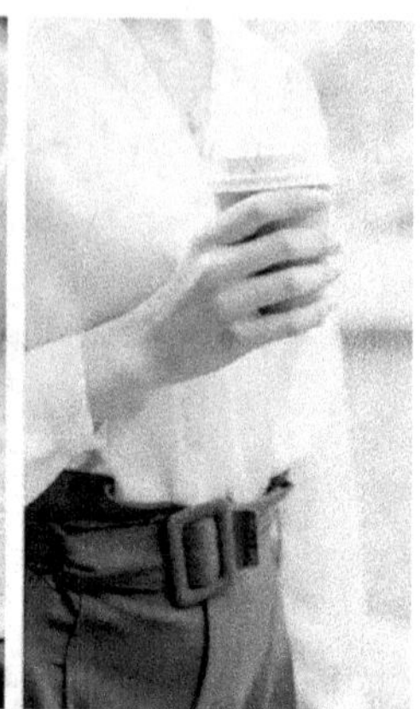

## First Signs: Hunger and Alcohol Loss

The transformation started with Intermittent Fasting (IF). At first, fasting for 24 hours was tough. It was confusing and difficult to manage. But after adjusting my window to something more sustainable; starting with morning lemon juice, apple cider vinegar, and coffee in the morning, and having my first meal at 7:00 PM. I noticed some profound changes.

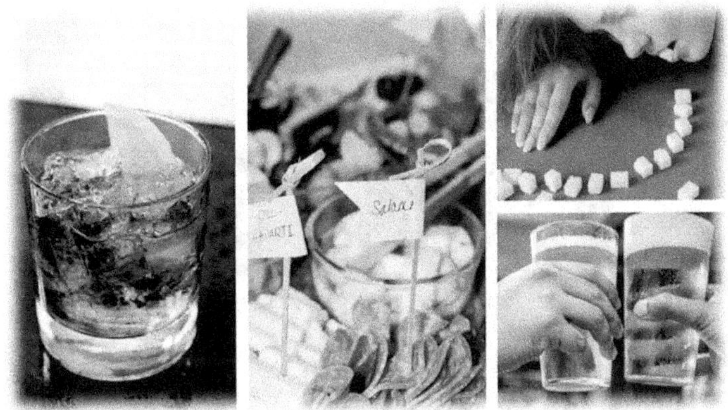

The most significant early change was that I lost the constant hunger I'd felt before. I no longer craved sugar or snacks throughout the day, and my desire for food seemed to diminish.

This new routine also had a surprising effect: I found that I simply no longer wanted alcohol. In the past, I would regularly drink, but when I tried to have a pint of beer after starting IF, it didn't taste as good as it once did. The craving was gone.

That moment was eye-opening. I realized that not only had I gained control over my hunger, but my body had begun rejecting things that weren't contributing to my well-being.

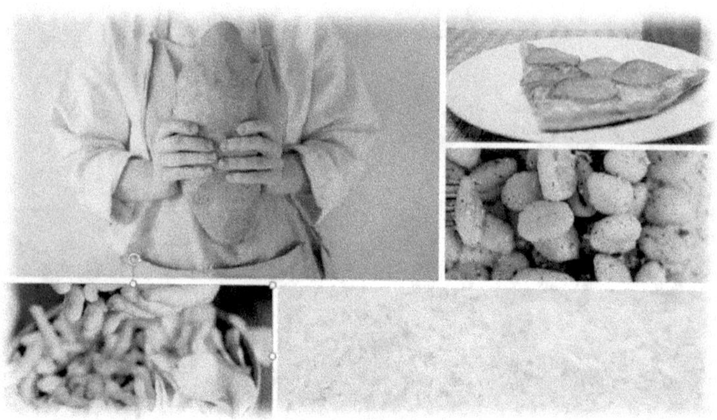

## Eliminating Sugar and Processed Foods

Along with IF, I made another crucial decision: I stopped consuming foods that I knew weren't serving my health.

This included cutting out sugar, rice, potatoes, pasta, bread, and white flour; all of which I had relied on as comfort foods in the past. I didn't miss them as much as I thought I would.

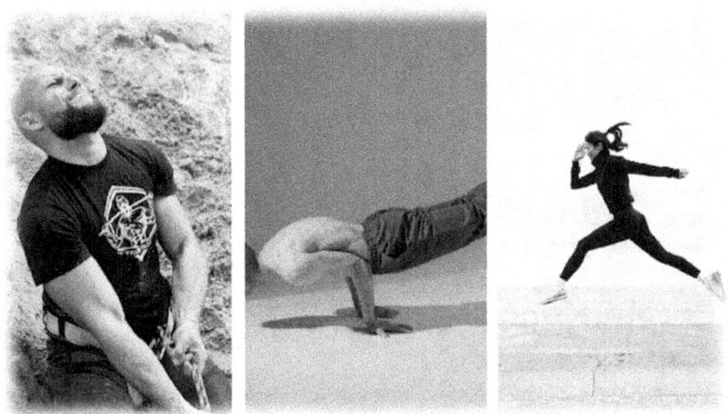

## Exercise – Moving Towards Health

This shift was powerful. Not only did my cravings for sugar and unhealthy foods decrease, but my energy levels increased, my blood sugar stabilized, and I felt clearer both mentally and physically.

4

# Chapter 4: Gaining Knowledge

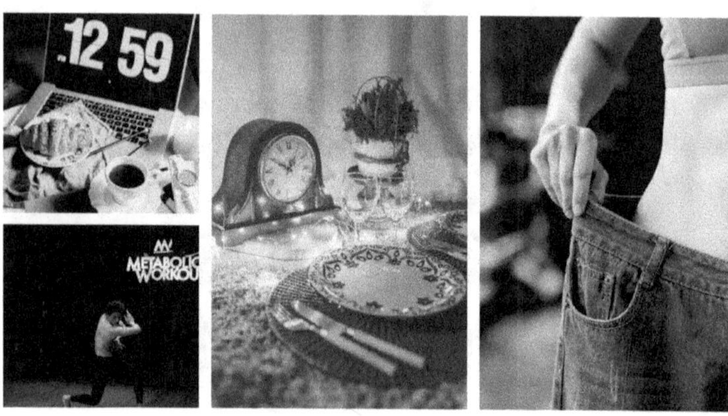

## How I Started with Intermittent Fasting (IF)

After deciding to take control of my health, I immersed myself in researching strategies to reverse Type 2 diabetes and enhance my overall well-being. One approach that immediately caught my attention was Intermittent Fasting (IF).

As I delved deeper into its benefits, I discovered that IF wasn't merely about skipping meals; it was a scientifically proven method to regulate blood sugar and promote fat loss. However, like any significant lifestyle change, I knew the key was to start gradually and find a routine that worked best for me.

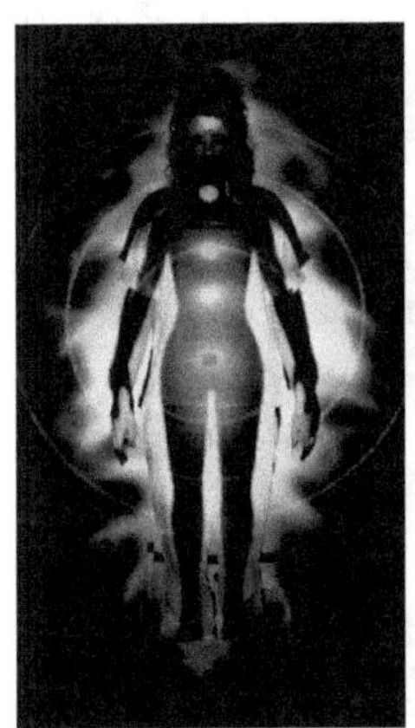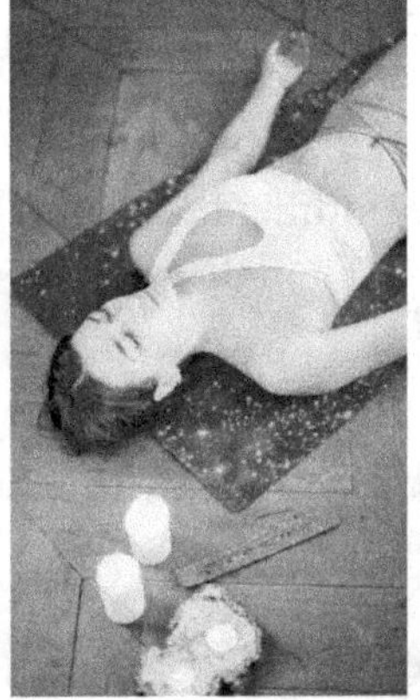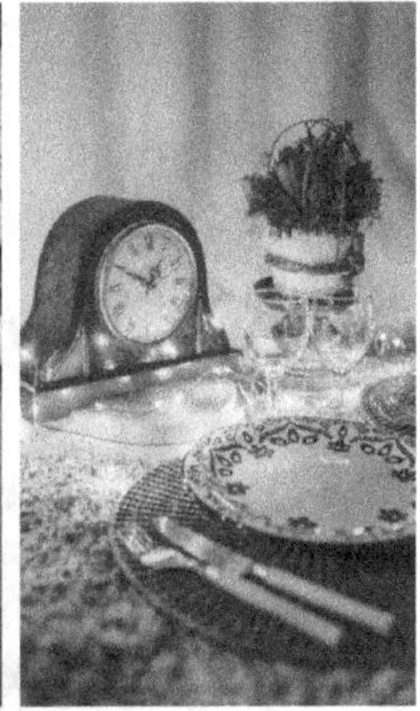

The first few days of intermittent fasting were tough. Going without food for extended hours felt uncomfortable, and there were moments of confusion about whether I was doing it right. But I soon realized that the key wasn't just about fasting; it was about understanding my body's signals and giving it the time and space it needed to heal.

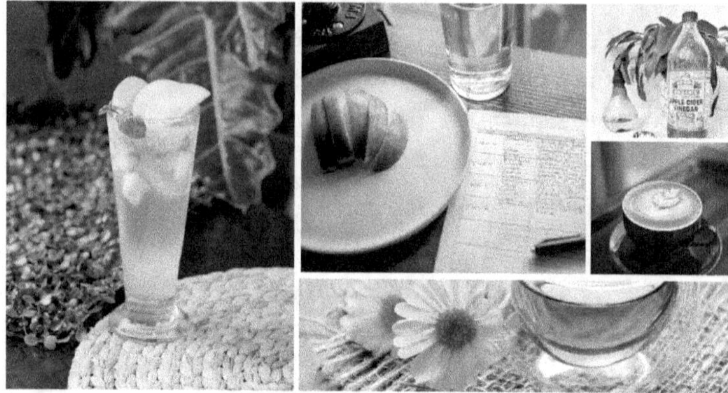

I chose to follow the 16:8 method. This meant fasting for 16 hours, with an 8-hour eating window. During the fasting period, I would have nothing but water, herbal teas, or black coffee to keep myself hydrated and curb any hunger.

I also introduced lemon water with apple cider vinegar in the morning to help with digestion and hydration.

Eating Window Schedule: 7:00 PM - 11:00 PM

| Time | Activity | Details |
| --- | --- | --- |
| 7:00 PM | Start of Eating Window | First meal of the day; light and nutritious dinner. |
| 8:00 PM | Family Time | Enjoying meals with family while maintaining the window. |
| 9:00 PM | Post-Meal Walk | Light 10 - 15-minute walk to aid digestion and regulate blood sugar. |
| 9:30 PM | Lighter Meals / Snacks | Gradual reduction in appetite; small, balanced snacks. |
| 10:00 PM | Slow Down | Mindful eating, preparing body for fasting again. |
| 11:00 PM | End of Eating Window | Final meal; no more eating after this time. |

My eating window was from 7:00 PM to 11:00 PM. At first, it was a little tricky adjusting to the idea of having my first meal so late in the evening, but I soon found it quite liberating.

This schedule worked well for me because it aligned with my natural routine and allowed me to enjoy dinner with family while still giving my body the time it needed to fast. I also noticed that I was not really eating a lot in my 8-hour eating window, as I gradually experienced a lack of appetite.

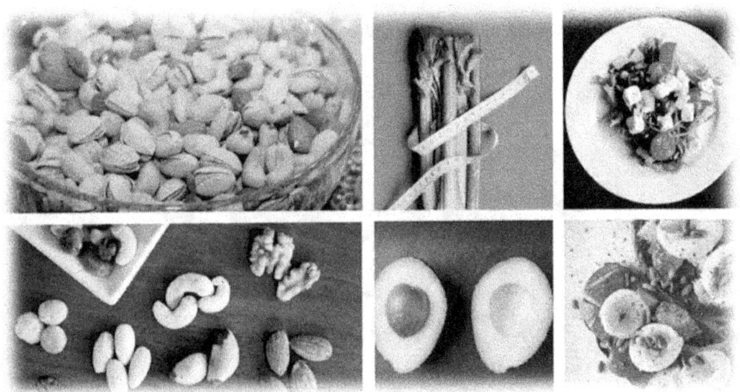

## Meal and Snack Details

My main meal, which I soon got accustomed to, was a satisfying and nutrient-packed dish consisting of Greek salad with feta cheese, eggs, avocado, celery, and a few other complementary ingredients. On alternate days, I would switch things up with another healthy variety of bio extras to keep things interesting and nutritious. Honestly, I often found myself unable to finish it all, as I felt full quite quickly due to the nutrient density of the meal.

At 9:30 PM, my snacks typically included a mix of almonds, walnuts, cashews, Brazil nuts, pistachios, hazelnuts, and a serving of Greek yogurt. These nutrient-dense options, paired with the natural sweetness of dates, made for an ideal snack, helping to maintain my energy levels and curb any remaining hunger before the fasting period started

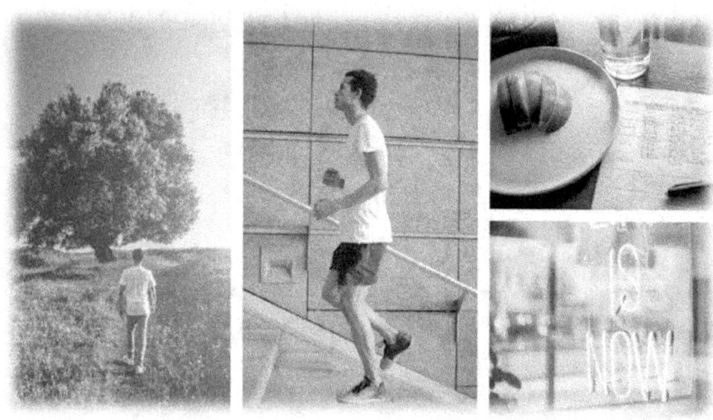

## Why Intermittent Fasting Worked for Me

Intermittent fasting didn't just help with weight loss; it became a lifestyle. What started out as a challenging task soon turned into a habit I couldn't imagine living without.  Fasting gave my digestive system the break it needed, and combined with walking and jogging, I began noticing improved mental clarity, increased energy, and better focus throughout the day.

These activities, alongside IF, not only helped regulate my blood sugar but also boosted my overall sense of well-being.

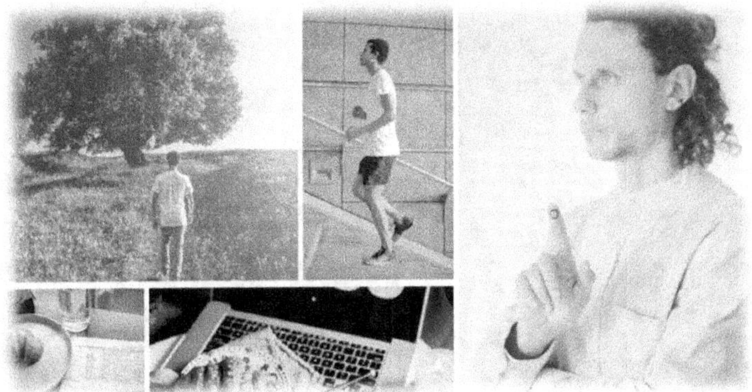

Even though I indulged in sugary treats like honey and dates, they never raised my blood sugar. This was thanks to the combination of burning more calories through IF, along with incorporating walking and jogging, which helped regulate my blood sugar levels and supported my overall health.

One of the best parts? It wasn't about restricting myself; it was about listening to my body and allowing it to function at its best. Eventually, IF became as natural as breathing. It was no longer just a "diet" or a "fad" – it evolved into an essential part of my daily routine, supporting both my health and my long-term goals.

**Other Intermittent Fasting Windows to Consider**

| Fasting Method | Fasting Duration | Eating Window | Benefits | Best For |
| --- | --- | --- | --- | --- |
| 16:8 Method | 16 hours | 8 hours | Simple, easy to follow, great for beginners; promotes fat loss, improves metabolism. | Beginners, those new to fasting |
| 18:6 Method | 18 hours | 6 Hours | Longer fast, accelerates fat loss, may improve insulin sensitivity. | Those looking for more fat loss benefits. |
| 20:4 Method | 20 hours | 4 hours | Advanced method for faster weight loss, enhanced insulin sensitivity | Experienced fasters, those seeking faster results |
| 5:2 Method | Eat normally 5 days | 2 fasting days | Flexible, allows regular meals most days, great for those who can't fast daily | Those looking for flexibility in fasting schedule |
| Eat-Stop-Eat Method | 24 hours (1-2x/week) | 24 hours (fast) | Extreme, can lead to significant health benefits, boosts fat loss. | Experienced fasters, those looking for extreme results. |

## *Important Note:*

Since everyone's body is different, it's important to understand that your system may process food differently than others. Therefore, before adopting any form of diet, exercise regimen, or intermittent fasting (IF), I strongly recommend consulting a healthcare professional. This ensures that the approach is right for your individual needs and health conditions.

## Integrating IF Part of My Life

What truly made intermittent fasting effective for me wasn't just the physical benefits; it was the ability to make it a sustainable part of my routine. As I tuned into my body's natural rhythm, I stopped feeling deprived and started feeling empowered. I also discovered that fasting sharpened my mental clarity, which was surprising because I had always believed eating was necessary for cognitive energy; especially with my demanding job.

The discipline I gained from IF extended beyond fasting; it positively impacted my exercise habits, mindfulness, and emotional health.

Keep in mind that there's no "one-size-fits-all" approach to intermittent fasting. The key is to listen to your body and adjust based on what feels right. The flexibility of IF allows it to evolve into an effortless and powerful tool that can improve your health over time.

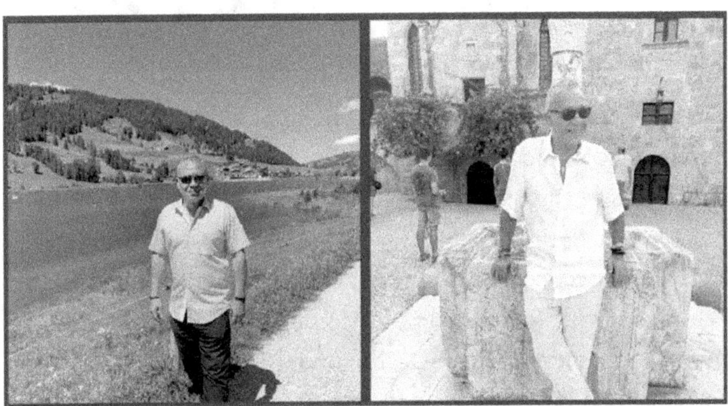

**My Transformation Journey: Before and After Intermittent Fasting**

**(LHS Picture 1- Before):** This image reflects the time when

I was struggling with energy, blood sugar issues, and overall health. At this stage, I was unaware of the changes I needed to make to improve my well-being.

**(RHS Picture 2- After):** This image represents the positive impact intermittent fasting had on my body and mind. I feel lighter, more energized, and mentally clearer than ever before.

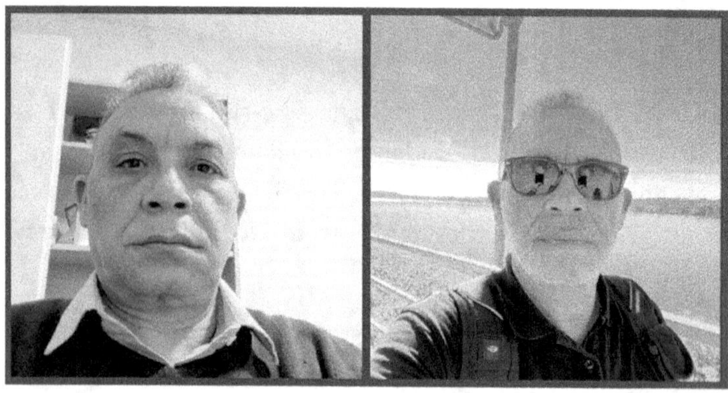

**(LHS Picture 3- Before):** I was facing bloating, tiredness, and feeling disconnected from my body. I knew something had to change but wasn't sure where to start.

**(RHS Picture 4- During Progress):** As I began intermittent fasting, I noticed a gradual reduction in weight and a significant increase in energy. This was the phase where I started seeing results and adjusting to the fasting windows.

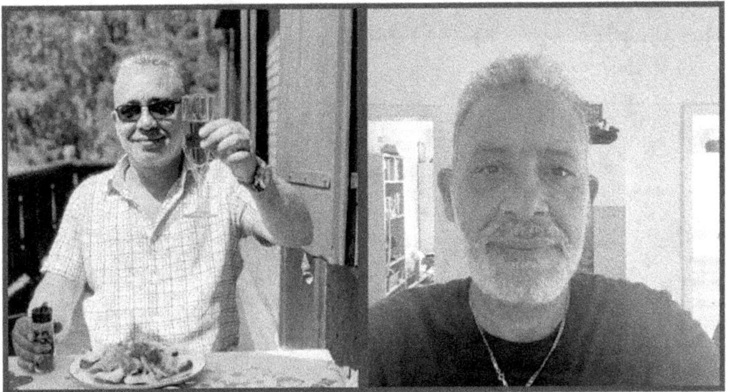

**(LHS Picture 5- Before):** This picture reflects a time when my diet and lifestyle choices weren't serving my health goals. I had become accustomed to indulging in alcohol and processed foods, which left me feeling sluggish, bloated, and low on energy.

**(RHS Picture 6- After):** This image represents the positive impact intermittent fasting had on my body and mind. I feel lighter, more energized, and experienced a newfound mental clarity.

## *Tracking Progress: Measuring Results*

| Week | Weight (kg) | Blood Sugar Level (mg/dL) | Notes |
| --- | --- | --- | --- |
| Week 1 | 90 kg | 130 mg/dL | Initial weight and higher blood sugar, starting the journey. |
| Week 2 | 88.5 kg | 120 mg/dL | Noticing some early changes, blood sugar starting to stabilize. |
| Week 3 | 86 kg | 110 mg/dL | Consistent progress, energy levels improving. |
| Week 4 | 84 kg | 105 mg/dL | Significant change, beginning to feel lighter and more energized. |
| Week 5 | 81.5 kg | 98 mg/dL | Weight loss continuing, blood sugar well under control. |
| Week 6 | 79 kg | 95 mg/dL | Accomplished steady progress, feeling much healthier and more motivated. |

It took me about 4 to 6 weeks to see the amazing results of my efforts. I was consistently measuring my blood sugar levels and weighing myself every morning.

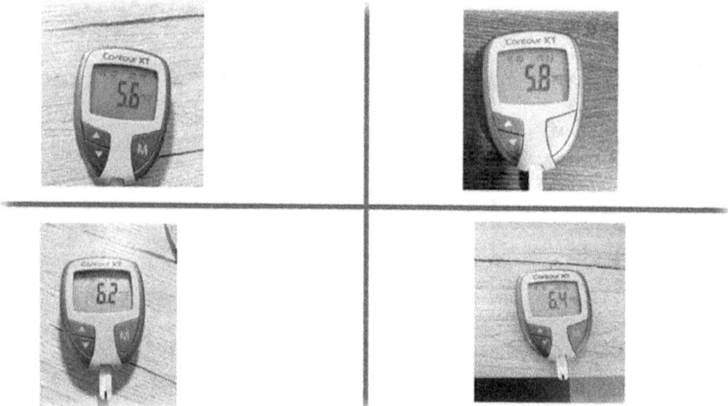

I was thrilled to see tangible results from my efforts as my weight steadily dropped and my blood sugar levels stabilized. My blood sugar readings consistently ranged between 5.6 and

6.4 mmol/L, which falls within the normal range.

These consistent improvements gave me a deep sense of accomplishment and reinforced my motivation to keep going. One of the most visible changes was the gradual disappearance of my beer belly, which had been a long-standing frustration.

The key to my success was consistency. By sticking to my healthy habits and staying dedicated, I saw steady progress each week. By the end of 6 weeks, I had achieved results that felt truly transformative. These changes proved that with determination and a clear plan, reaching my target weight of 69 kg was entirely achievable.

On average, I lost approximately 0.25–0.3 kg (0.5–0.66 lbs) per day through intermittent fasting, light exercise like walking, and mindful eating. Over 6 weeks, this added up to an impressive total of 11 kg (24 lbs). Achieving this level of progress required a medium level of effort; manageable for anyone who remains consistent and listens to their body.

This journey wasn't just about losing weight; it was about reclaiming my health, energy, and overall well-being. It's proof that small, sustainable changes can lead to significant transformations.

5

# Chapter 5: Overcoming Setbacks

**F**acing the Challenges Head-On

Embarking on a journey to improve my health was no easy feat. Along the way, I encountered a series of challenges that tested my resolve. From physical hurdles to emotional struggles, every step forward seemed to be met with another obstacle. But with each setback, I grew more determined to push through and keep going. Staying motivated wasn't always easy, but I discovered several key strategies that helped me maintain focus, even when things felt tough.

## Facing Obstacles

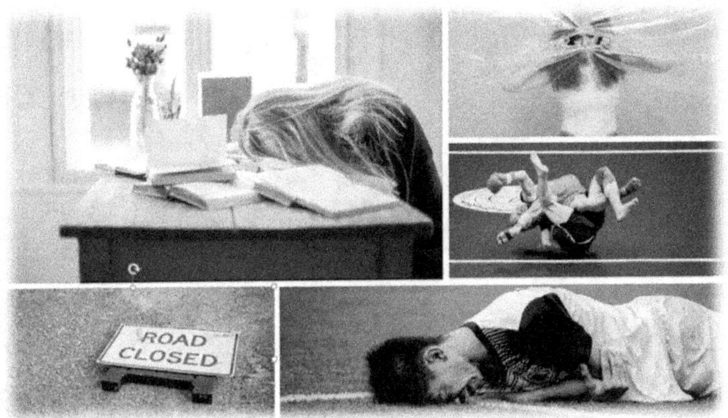


One of the biggest challenges I faced was dealing with the physical limitations that came with being overweight and having Type 2 diabetes. Fatigue, difficulty starting exercise, and the constant battle against unhealthy cravings were all roadblocks that could have easily discouraged me. On top of this, the emotional weight of my diagnosis was a constant reminder of what was at stake.

However, the most difficult obstacle was procrastination. As I struggled with my health, I found myself putting off tasks that were essential, like sticking to my diet, exercising regularly, and even learning more about my condition. Procrastination became a barrier to my progress, and I knew overcoming it was key to making real change.

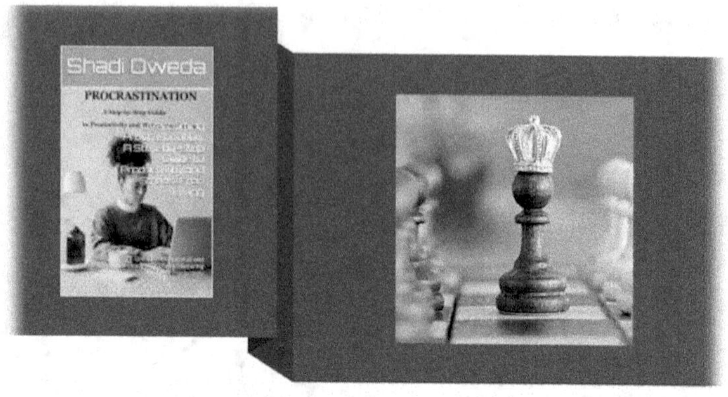

In my book Overcoming Procrastination: *[A **Step-by-Step
Guide to Productivity and Stress-Free Living**]*, I explore how
procrastination not only affects our productivity but also
undermines our well-being. The strategies I discussed, such as
breaking tasks into smaller, manageable steps, were essential
in helping me tackle procrastination in my health journey.
By focusing on one task at a time, I gradually overcame
procrastination and started making real progress.

## Mindset Shifts

I also had to work hard on changing my mindset. There
were days when it felt like the journey was too difficult, and
I questioned if I could ever truly overcome the health issues I
was facing. But I learned that setbacks weren't failures; they
were simply part of the journey. Instead of seeing challenges as
obstacles that could derail my progress, I began to view them
as opportunities to learn and grow.

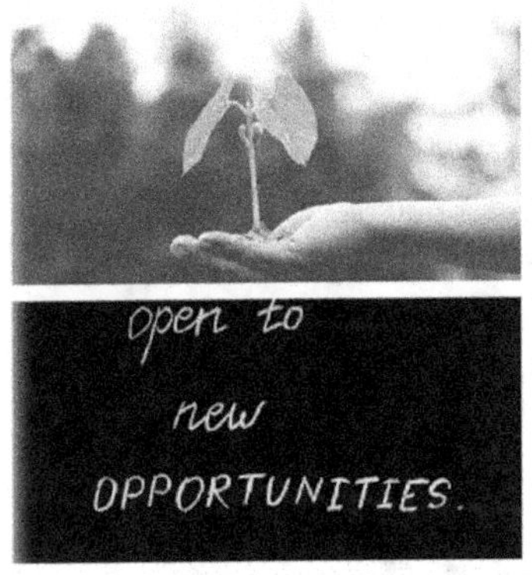


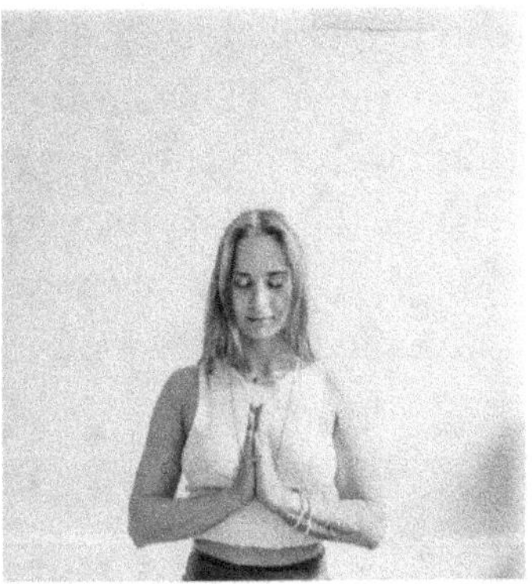

This shift in mindset allowed me to approach each setback with a sense of resilience. I learned to embrace the discomfort of change, knowing that it would lead to long-term rewards. Each time I stumbled, I reminded myself that these moments were not signs of failure—they were signs of progress.

## Staying Focused

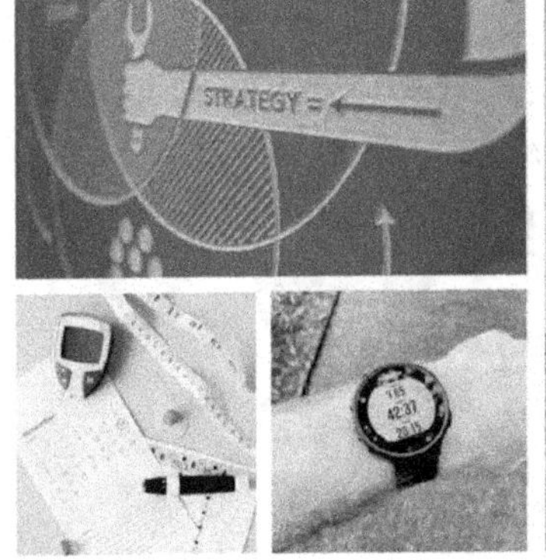


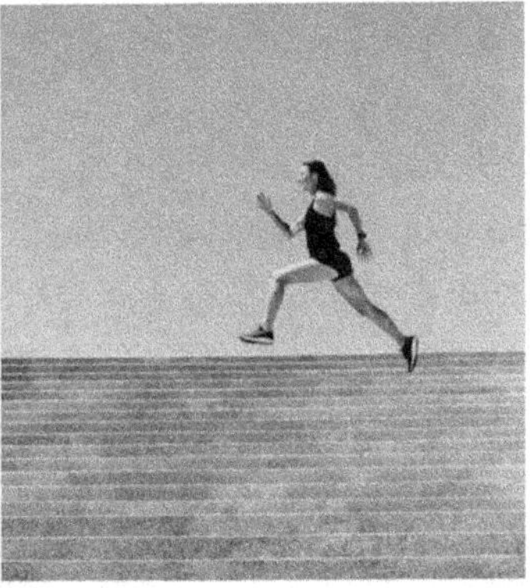

On tough days, when motivation seemed elusive, I turned to

the strategies that had helped me make progress in the first place. I focused on the small victories. I reminded myself of the results I was seeing: the weight loss, the improved blood sugar levels, and the way my energy levels had skyrocketed. I tracked my weight and blood sugar every day, and each positive change was a reminder of why I was doing this.

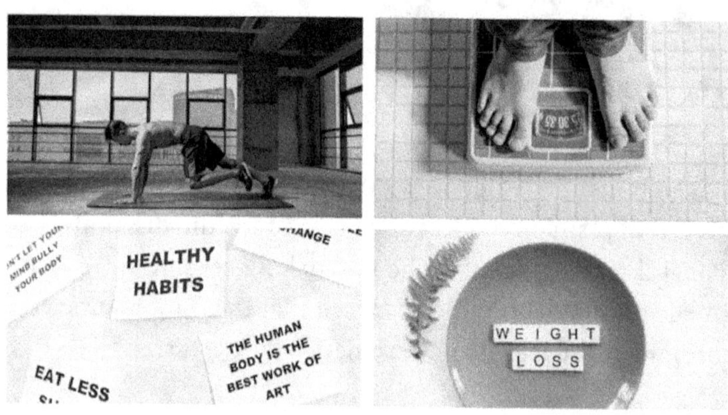


For example, when I started, my goal was to reduce my weight from 90kg to 69kg, which the BMI calculator indicated as my ideal weight range. I recorded my weight every morning without clothes, as well as after each workout session. The more I pushed myself to stay active, the more impressive the results became.

## Support Systems

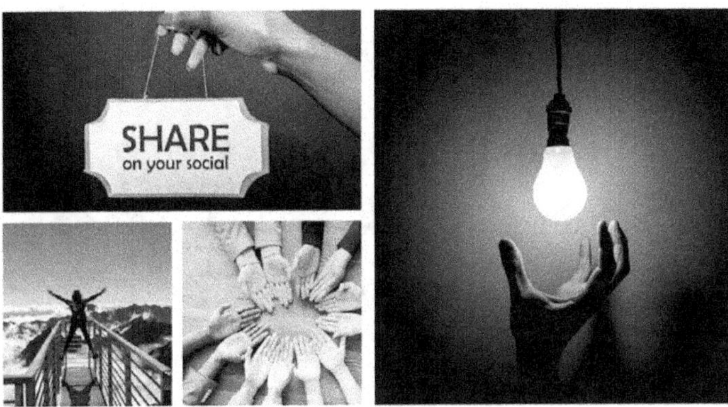


Throughout my journey, I leaned heavily on the support of those around me. My family played an instrumental role in keeping me motivated, providing encouragement, and celebrating my victories. Additionally, online communities where people were experiencing similar challenges became a source of strength. The connections I made with others striving for better health helped me feel less isolated and reminded me I wasn't alone.

6

# Chapter 6: A Change in Diet and Routine

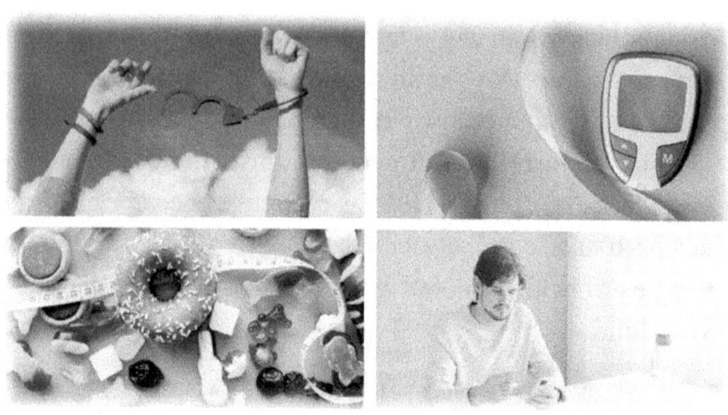

## Why I Needed a Change

When I first received my Type 2 diabetes diagnosis, I knew that something had to change. I had spent years neglecting my health and relying on convenience foods that were easy to grab but far from beneficial. My blood sugar levels were high, my energy was low, and I felt trapped in a cycle of poor habits. It became clear to me that reversing Type 2 diabetes wasn't just about medication or momentary changes; it was about completely overhauling my lifestyle, particularly my diet.

I needed a new routine that would nourish my body, support my blood sugar levels, and provide the energy I so desperately lacked.

## Diet and Exercise Changes

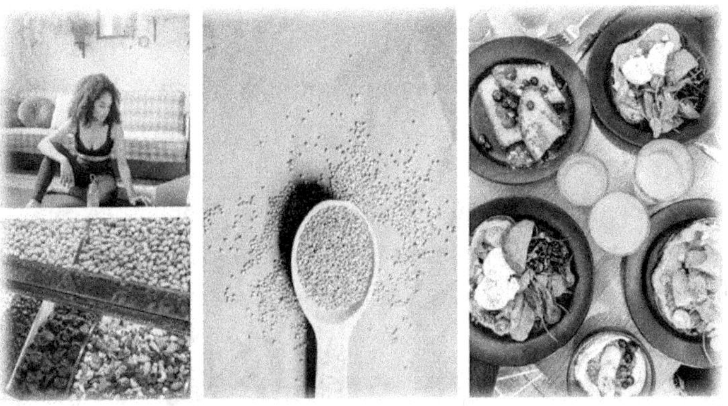

The first major shift I made was with my diet. I became incredibly selective about what I put into my body. I didn't just want to eat food; I wanted food that would fuel me, support my body's needs, and help me reverse my diabetes.

I started focusing on nutrient-dense foods that provided the necessary vitamins and minerals my body needed to function optimally.

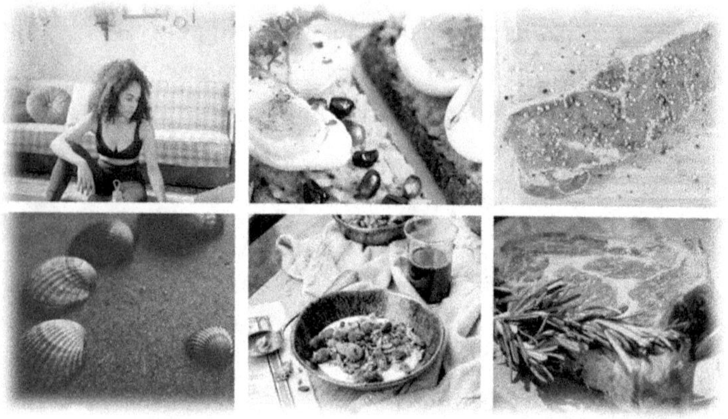

For example, I made sure to include plenty of B12-rich foods such as meat, eggs, and fortified cereals. These are essential for nerve function and energy production, which were both critical in my journey.

I also increased my intake of leafy green vegetables like spinach and kale, which are packed with essential vitamins, fiber, and antioxidants that support healthy blood sugar levels.

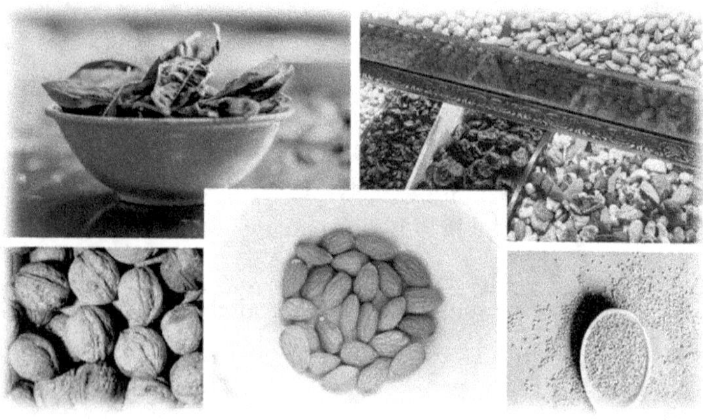

Nuts, including walnuts, and cashews, became a staple in my diet as well. Packed with healthy fats, protein, and fiber, they helped keep me full and satisfied, while also providing magnesium, which is essential for blood sugar regulation.

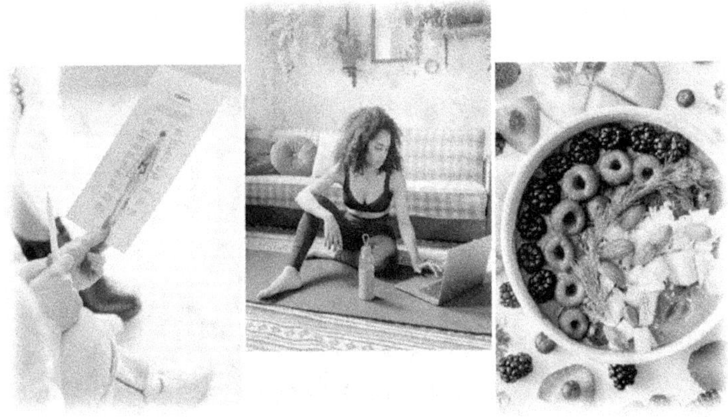

I added more berries to my meals—blueberries, strawberries, and raspberries; as they are rich in antioxidants and have a low glycemic index, making them ideal for a diabetic-friendly diet.

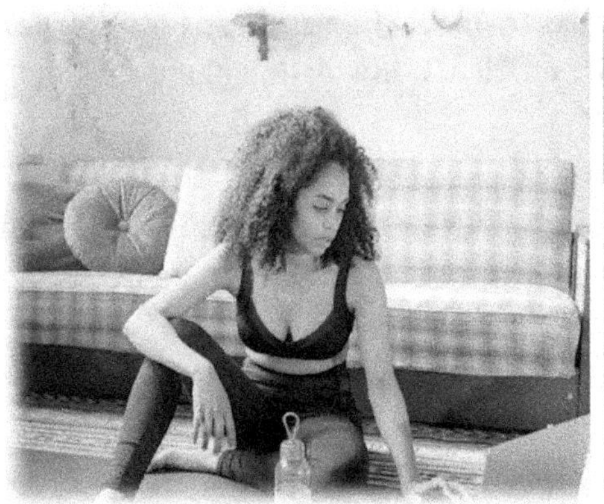
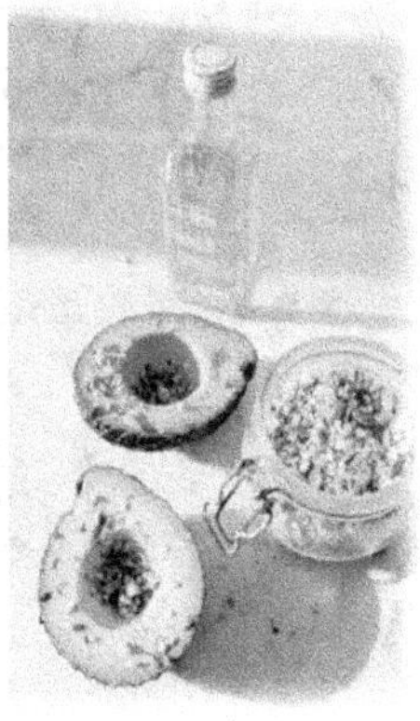

I also incorporated healthy fats such as olive oil and avocado into my meals. These fats helped reduce inflammation in my body and kept me feeling full longer. I became intentional with my food choices, always thinking about how each meal could nourish my body, regulate my blood sugar, and support my health.

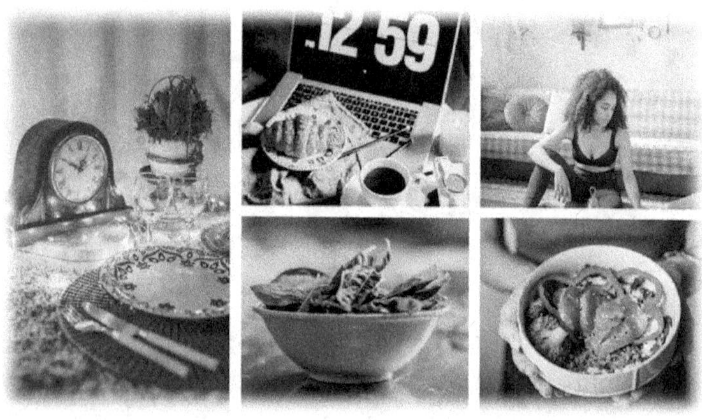

In addition to my diet, I restructured my eating schedule. I followed intermittent fasting, giving my body time to rest and recover between meals. By fasting for a set period each day, my body became more efficient at regulating blood sugar and burning fat.

I also made sure to eat foods with a to avoid spikes in blood sugar and help my body better manage insulin levels.

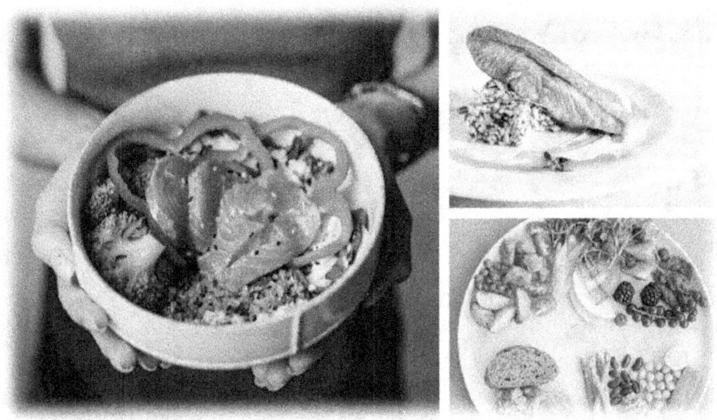

Alongside these dietary changes, I knew that exercise would play a crucial role in my journey. So, I began to exercise regularly, starting with simple routines and gradually increasing the intensity.

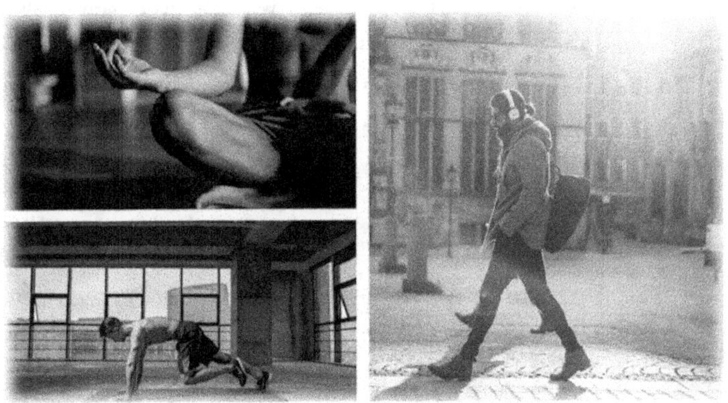

*At first, I focused on building up my strength and endurance with light walking and resistance exercises. These helped me increase my muscle mass and improve my insulin sensitivity.*

## The Power of Walking

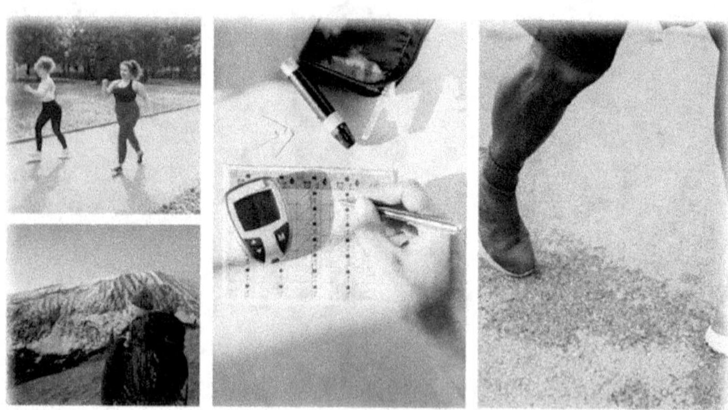

Walking, although simple, became an essential part of my daily routine. It was one of the most effective exercises I could do to help control my blood sugar levels. I started walking every day; at first, it was just a 10-minute walk around the block. Over time, I increased the duration and intensity, adding brisk walking and hill walking to challenge myself further. Walking became more than just a way to get in shape; it was a powerful tool in controlling my blood sugar.

Walking helped lower my blood sugar levels in several ways: it improved my insulin sensitivity, increased blood circulation, and helped burn fat. What made it so effective was the fact that it didn't feel like a burden or a complicated exercise routine. It was something I could do daily without a lot of effort, and it was easy to incorporate into my schedule. Even on busy days, a simple walk was enough to keep my health on track. I also noticed that after each walk, when dopamine was released, I felt a sense of happiness and well-being. This positive feeling kept me motivated, and I stuck to my routine, knowing how beneficial it was for both my physical and emotional health.

## The Importance of Consistency

As I continued making these changes, I realized that consistency was key. It wasn't enough to eat healthy or exercise occasionally. I had to commit to a new routine, one that I could maintain in the long run. Every single day became an opportunity to strengthen my resolve and work towards my goal of reversing Type 2 diabetes. Maintaining a consistent diet, exercise routine, and fasting schedule helped me stay focused and kept me on the path to better health.

I created small, sustainable habits that built upon one another, and soon, they became second nature. For example, I no longer had to remind myself to eat healthier; it became a part of my lifestyle. Similarly, my daily walks became a regular part of my day, something I looked forward to rather than a chore.

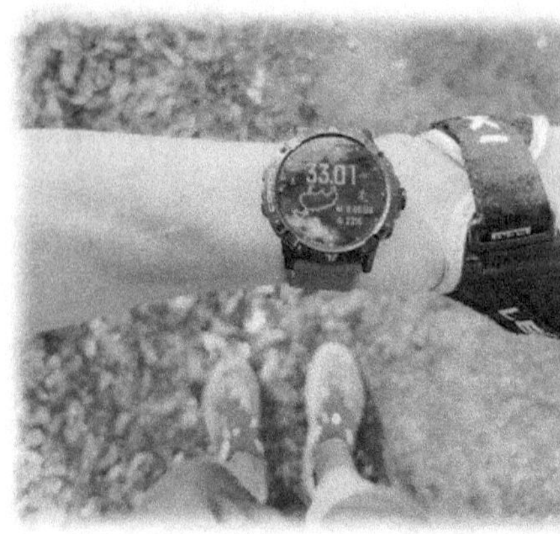
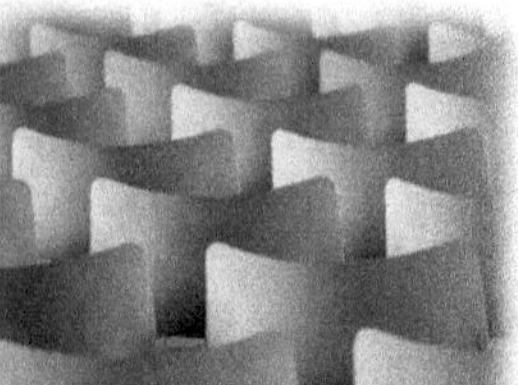
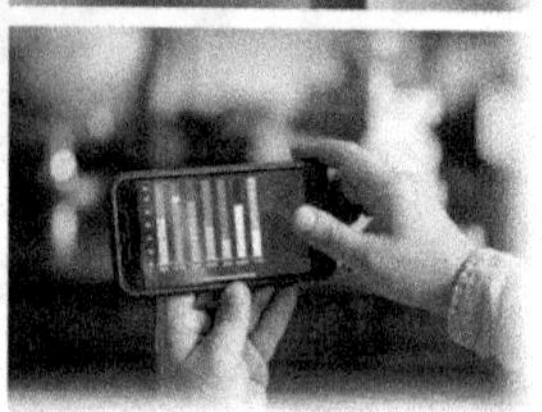

I also noticed the power of consistency in tracking my progress. Each week, I would measure my blood sugar levels, weigh myself, and record any other changes. I could see how my hard work was paying off, and that kept me motivated to keep going. The more consistent I was with my new routine, the more positive results I saw.

What I learned along the way was that the changes I made weren't just temporary fixes—they were lifestyle changes that would support my health for years to come. By committing to a consistent routine of healthy eating, exercise, and intermittent fasting, I was setting myself up for long-term success.

# 7

# Chapter 7: The Role of Mindfulness

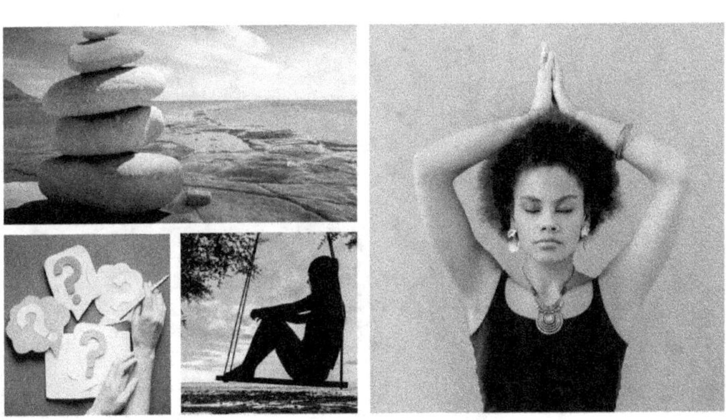

# How Mental Awareness Enhanced My Physical Transformation

As I continued my journey toward better health and reversing Type 2 diabetes, I realized that my transformation was not only about diet and exercise. It was about how I tuned into my body and mind. The physical changes I was experiencing were powerful, but they were complemented by a deeper mental shift; one that helped me gain a clearer understanding of my emotions, cravings, and behaviors.

For many years, I had ignored the signals my body sent me. Stress, distractions, and a lack of awareness kept me focused on external goals like weight loss and blood sugar control. I rarely paused to check in with how I was truly feeling; both physically and mentally.

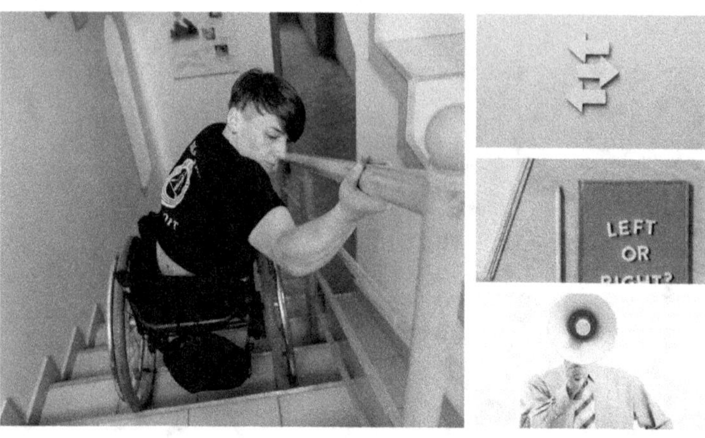


When I began incorporating mindfulness into my routine, it was a revelation. While exercise and a healthy diet were the cornerstones of my physical transformation, mindfulness became the mental exercise that helped me navigate challenges, stay grounded, and make better choices. It taught me to pay attention to my body's cues without judgment or rush.

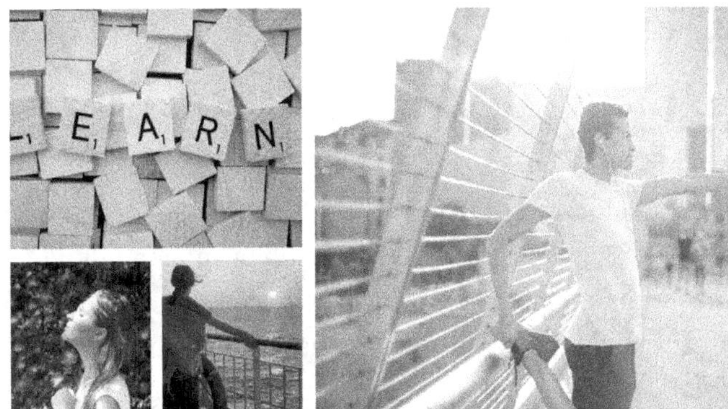

Mindfulness wasn't about following a rigid routine or trying to achieve specific outcomes. It was about learning to tune into what my body and mind were communicating in the present moment. It gave me the space to slow down and truly listen to myself, helping me make choices that were more aligned with my health goals.

## The Mental Shift

In light of the changes I experienced, I noticed a shift in my relationship with hunger.  Rather than the usual cravings, I found myself more in control. When fatigue set in, I recognized the need to rest. I no longer felt the familiar hunger, but when my body signaled for nourishment, I became more attuned to what it truly needed, choosing wholesome foods over the old habit of reaching for unhealthy snacks. This mental shift, coupled with my physical efforts, empowered me to cultivate a healthier, more sustainable lifestyle.

# 8

# Chapter 8: Measuring My Success

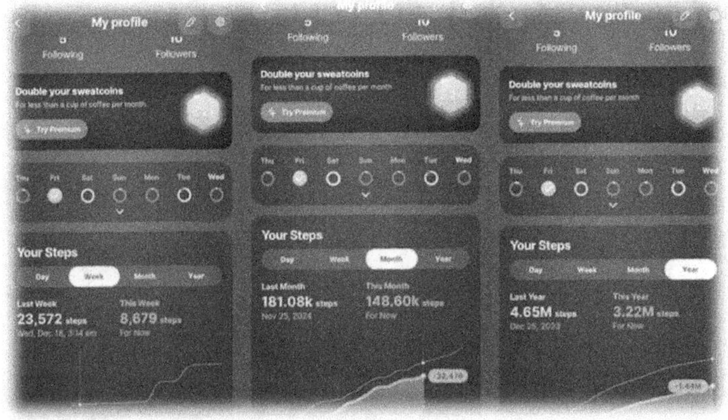

## Why Tracking Matters

When walking and hitting my daily milestones, I often felt a sense of achievement that only I knew about, especially when I walked alone. This sense of accomplishment was enough for me until I discovered apps like Sweatcoin and Macadam.

These apps quickly became valuable companions on my walks, rewarding me with coins and cash for the distance I covered. The rewards were motivating, but what I found most exciting was how they added a fun, competitive element to my routine.

As I continued using these apps, I began collecting coins and cash, which made the experience even more engaging. I even entered challenges, one of which was to walk 250K steps in one month to support a charity for water in Africa. To my delight, I surpassed the goal and reached 500K steps, which was an accomplishment I was proud of. This added another layer of motivation, reinforcing the importance of tracking my success in different ways.

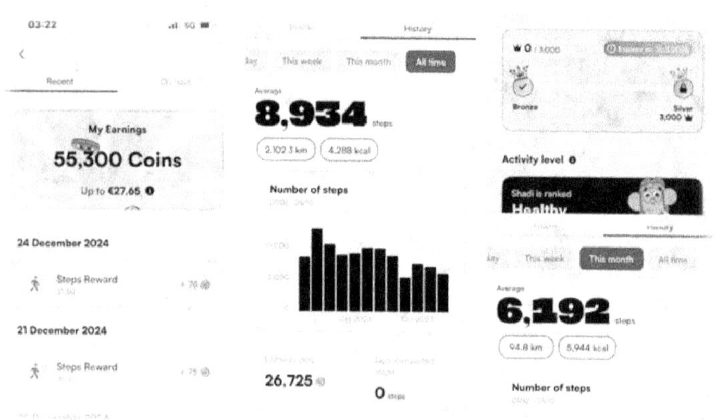

One of the most empowering parts of my journey to reverse Type 2 diabetes was seeing tangible evidence of my progress. Monitoring my blood sugar levels and weight became a powerful motivator, allowing me to track the improvements I was making in real-time. Each drop in my blood sugar or weight felt like a victory, a confirmation that my efforts were paying off. For someone who had been living with diabetes for so long, these small changes were huge milestones, and they kept me focused on my goal of reclaiming my health.

Tracking gave me the ability to stay accountable and understand how my lifestyle choices were impacting my body. It allowed me to adjust my diet, exercise, and overall approach, making the journey feel less uncertain and more within my control. It was no longer just about hoping things would improve; it was about watching real-time results unfold, which motivated me to keep pushing forward.

*[As part of the growing trend of fitness apps and wristbands that encourage walking, two popular options include SweatCoin (available at www.sweatco.in) and Macadam (downloadable from the Google Play Store or Apple App Store). Additionally, Mi Fit (by Xiaomi) can also be downloaded from the Google Play Store or Apple App Store.]*

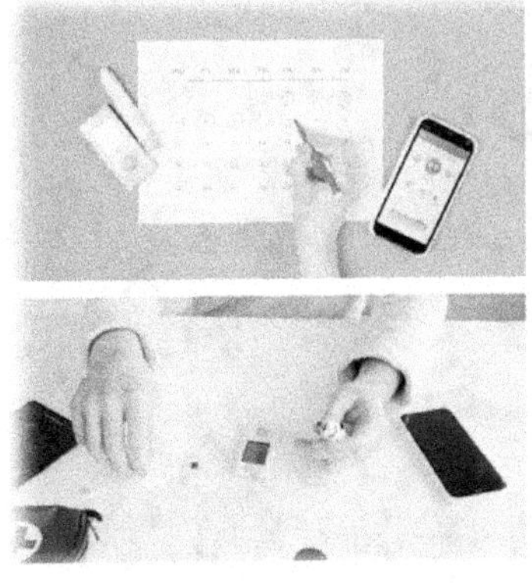
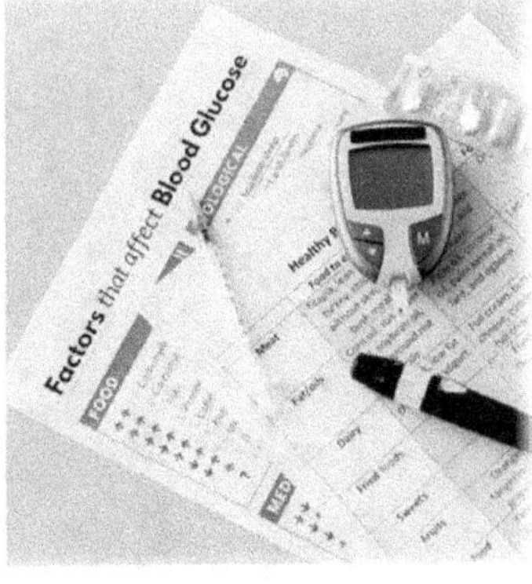

## Tools and Techniques for Tracking

To stay on track in my journey, I relied on various tools
to monitor my progress. Apps and fitness trackers became
essential in my daily routine.

Blood sugar monitoring apps made it easy to log readings and
analyze trends. They not only tracked my blood sugar but also
provided insights into how my food, stress, and activity levels
impacted it. Weight tracking apps helped me log my weight,
giving me instant motivation as I saw numbers drop over time.

I combined these apps with fitness bands that tracked my
daily steps, calories burned, and overall physical activity. They
encouraged me to meet daily goals and helped me correlate my
exercise with improvements in blood sugar and weight.

Having these tools made my journey more data driven. I could
see clear patterns in my health metrics, and the data gave me
confidence that the changes I was making were effective.

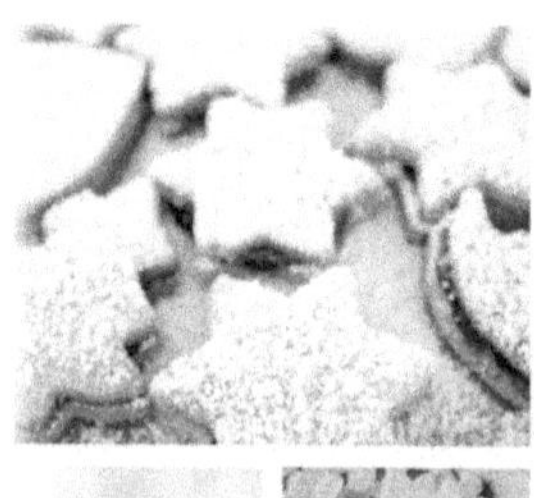
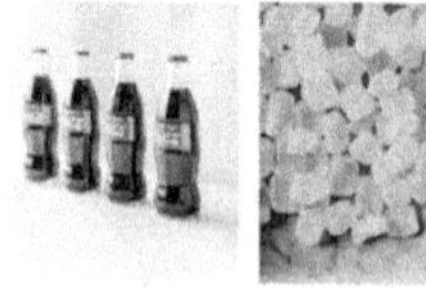
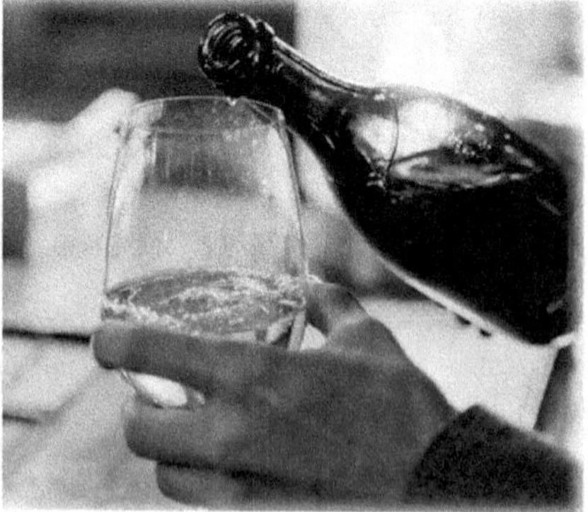

## Adjusting Based on Data

Tracking also allowed me to make adjustments based on real-time data. For example, when certain foods caused blood sugar spikes, I could replace them with healthier options. If my weight loss plateaued, I could fine-tune my routine to keep moving forward.

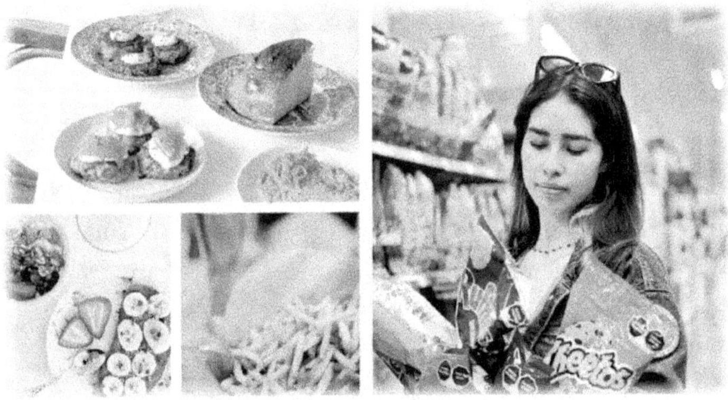

This personalized approach empowered me. Instead of being discouraged by fluctuations, I used them as opportunities to tweak my plan and avoid setbacks. It was like having a roadmap that helped me stay on course.

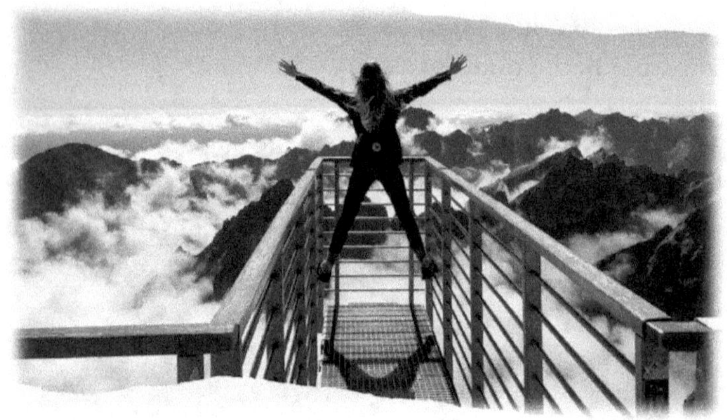

## Celebrating Milestones

Tracking wasn't just about data; it was about celebrating victories. Each time my blood sugar dropped into the normal range, or I saw the scale move down, it reinforced my commitment to my health.

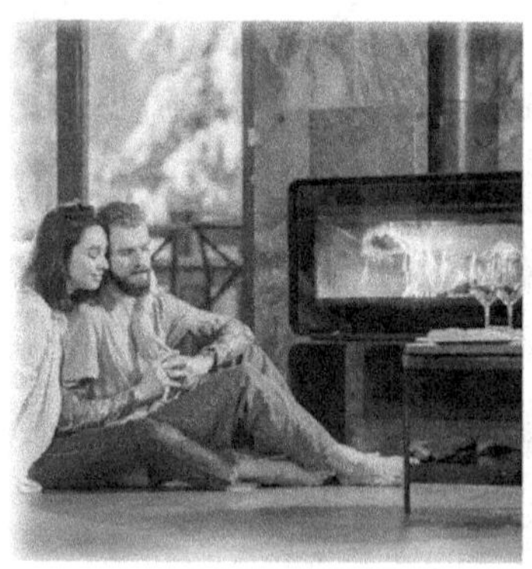
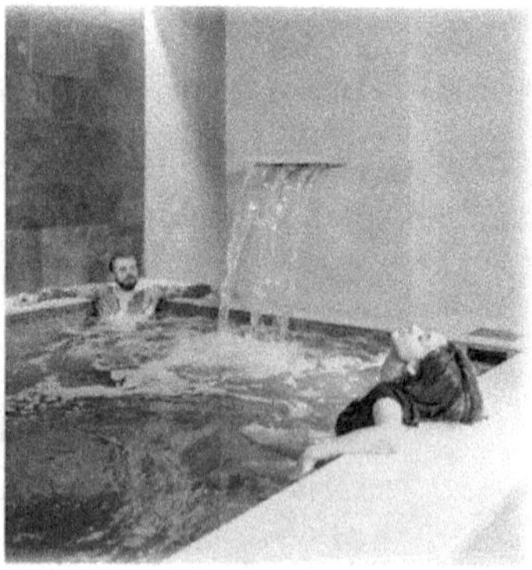

I celebrated these milestones with healthy treats, a day off to relax, or simply reflecting on my progress. Every small victory reminded me that the journey to better health was about both the long-term goal and the incremental successes along the way.

Tracking showed me that success isn't always linear. Some days were slower than others but knowing that I was making progress kept me motivated. Each milestone, no matter how small, reminded me of the power of persistence and self-care.

9

# Chapter 9: Sustainable Habits

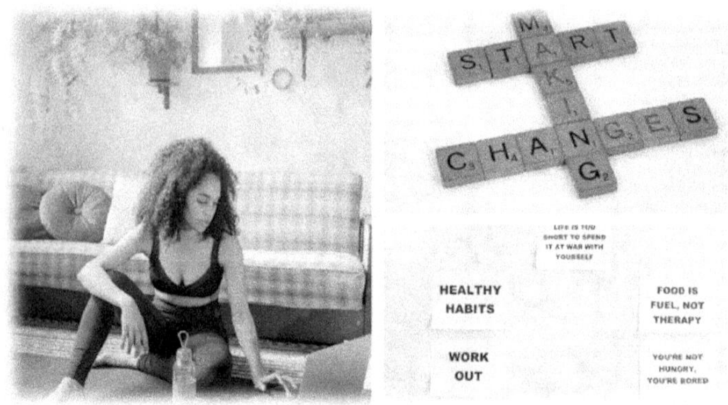


**uilding Lasting Habits**

B Long-term health success isn't about short-term diets or quick fixes; it's about building sustainable habits. Small, incremental changes that fit seamlessly into daily life made all the difference for me.

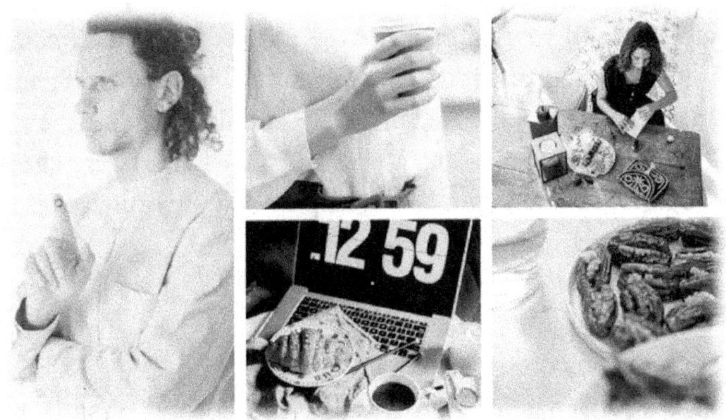

One of the most transformative habits I adopted was intermittent fasting. Initially, it felt challenging, but it soon became part of my routine, giving my body time to rest and reset.

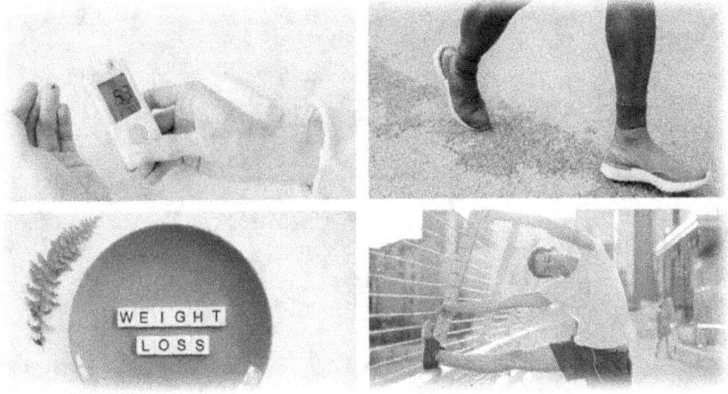


Daily walking was another essential habit, providing physical activity that was easy to integrate into my life. Together, these practices became non-negotiable priorities, leading to better blood sugar control, weight loss, and improved mental clarity.

I also learned to avoid quick fixes. Fad diets and extreme solutions might offer immediate results, but they aren't sustainable. Instead, I focused on small, meaningful adjustments; modifying my diet, staying active, and managing stress. These changes brought gradual, lasting improvements without feeling overwhelmed.

Consistency, not perfection, became my mantra. Occasional slip-ups didn't derail my progress because I focused on showing up daily and staying on course. Over time, these habits became automatic; a natural part of who I am.

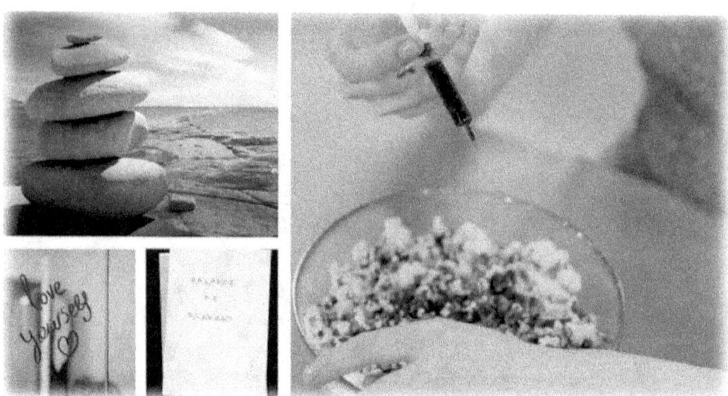

As my journey evolved, I adapted my routine to meet my changing needs, from experimenting with new foods to finding better ways to stay motivated. I also prioritized mental health through mindfulness, stress management, and self-care, ensuring balance and emotional wellbeing. These simple yet powerful habits-fasting, walking, eating well; became the foundation of my lifestyle. They've helped me maintain my health and remain a part of my life for the long term.

61

10

# Chapter 10: The Emotional Journey

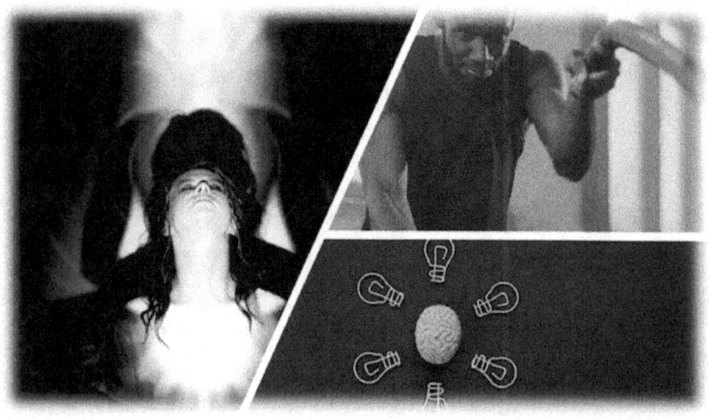

**Healing Beyond the Physical**

My journey to better health wasn't just about physical changes; it transformed me emotionally, mentally, and spiritually. Losing weight and managing Type 2 diabetes lifted not only the physical burden but also the emotional weight I'd been carrying. I felt lighter, more balanced, and revitalized in every sense.

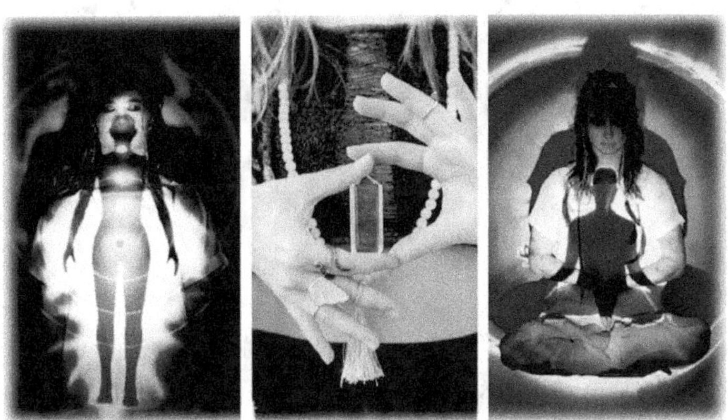

## The Emotional Side of Healing

I realized that physical health and emotional wellbeing are deeply connected. Years of frustration and fear around my diagnosis had taken an emotional toll. As my body healed, so did my mind. Letting go of this emotional baggage was just as important as addressing my diet and exercise habits.

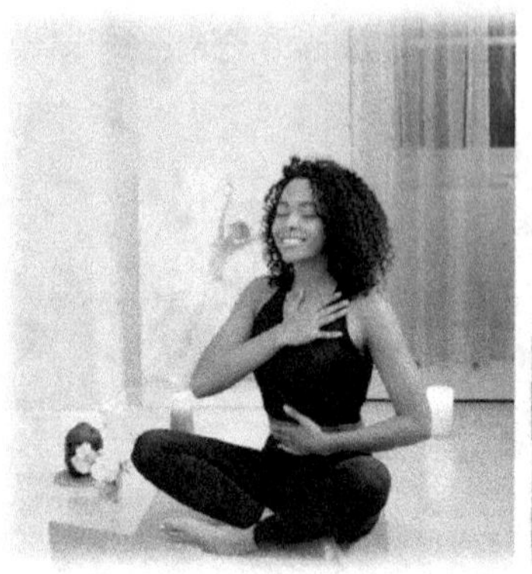
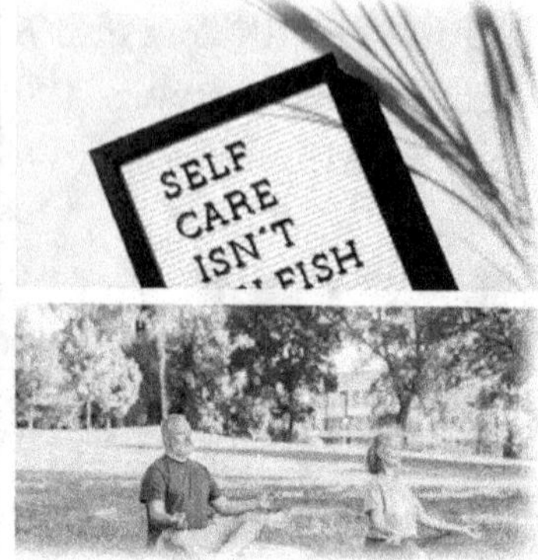


## Managing Stress

Stress often derailed my progress, but I learned to manage it
through mindfulness, deep breathing, and meditation. Self-
care became a priority, whether it was spending time in nature,
resting, or engaging in joyful activities. Lowering stress
improved not only my emotional balance but also my overall
health.

## Emotional Growth

This journey forced me to confront self-doubt and negativity.
By fostering resilience and a positive mindset, I began to heal
from within. I stopped tying my worth to numbers like weight
or blood sugar levels and instead focused on emotional growth
and progress.

## Self-Care and Self-Love

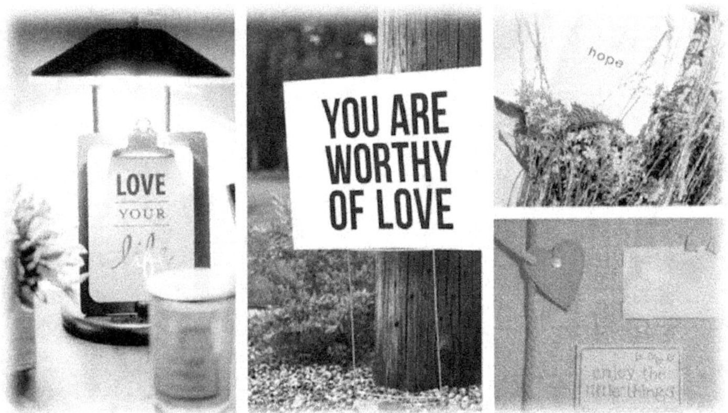


Compassion for myself became vital. I let go of perfectionism and embraced my wins, no matter how small. Self-care—like taking walks, reading, or connecting with loved ones, nourished me. I learned to listen to my body and honor its needs, building a foundation of self-love that sustained my transformation. Through emotional healing, stress management, and self-care, I created a life that felt lighter, more purposeful, and fulfilling. This inner growth was the key to sustaining my health and embracing the future with hope.

<br>

11

# Chapter 11: The Transformative Power of Restorative Sleep

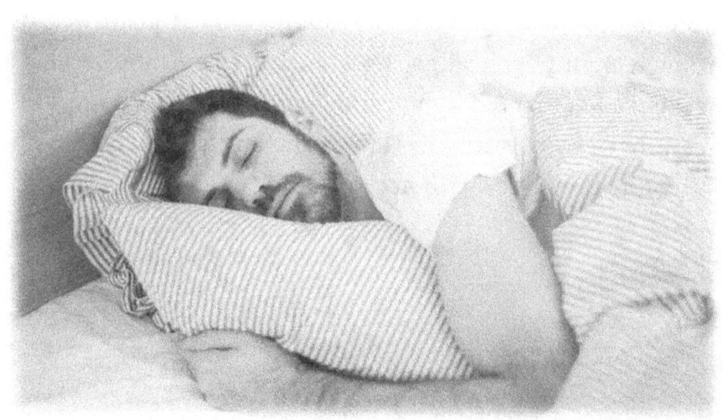

## Why Sleep Matters

Sleep is essential for health, especially in managing Type 2 diabetes and weight loss. During deep sleep, the body repairs itself, regulates insulin, and balances hormones. Poor sleep disrupts these processes, leading to higher blood sugar, cravings, and low energy.

Once I prioritized restorative sleep, I noticed improved energy, stress management, and progress in reversing diabetes and losing weight.

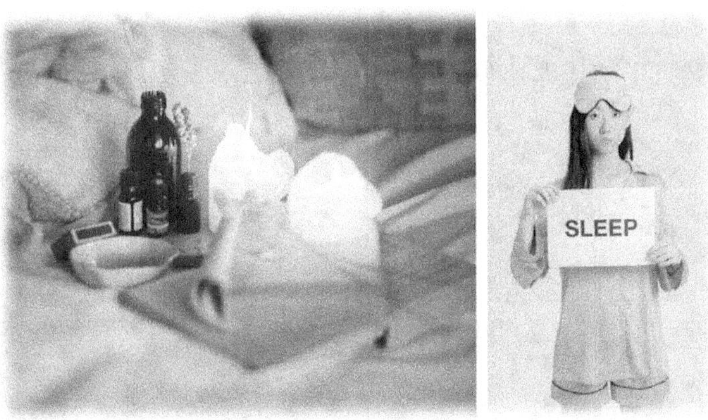


## Improving Sleep Habits

One of the most impactful lifestyle changes I made was enhancing my sleep routine. I adopted a consistent sleep schedule, optimized my bedroom environment (cool, dark, and quiet), and eliminated distractions like electronics. These changes boosted my energy, enabling me to stay consistent with exercise and healthier habits. Emotionally, I felt more balanced and less irritable.

## Sleep and Stress

Stress had been a major obstacle in my health journey. Poor sleep exacerbated my anxiety and made diabetes management harder. However, once I improved my sleep, my ability to handle stress improved significantly. Restful nights left me feeling refreshed and resilient, allowing me to approach setbacks with clarity and positivity.

## Tips for Better Sleep

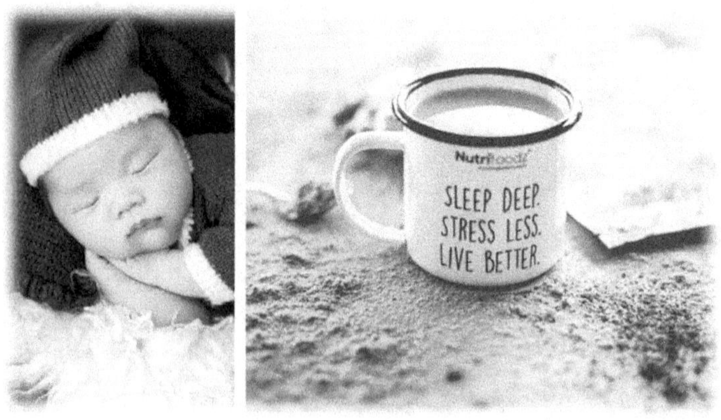


**Here are strategies that transformed my sleep:**

**Reduce Screen Time:** Avoid electronics 30 minutes before bed.

**Establish a Routine:** Relaxing activities like reading or deep breathing signal your body to wind down.

**Create a Restful Environment:** Keep your bedroom cool, dark, and quiet; invest in blackout curtains and white noise.

**Manage Stress During the Day:** Mindfulness and avoiding caffeine or heavy meals late in the day improve sleep quality.

**Be Consistent:** Stick to the same sleep and wake times daily to regulate your cycle. By following these practices, sleep became a cornerstone of my health journey. It not only improved my physical wellbeing but also enhanced my emotional and mental balance. Restorative sleep gave me the energy and focus to face challenges and stay on the path to healing.

# 12

# Chapter 12: Reflecting on My Transformation

**L**ooking Back, Moving Forward

As I reflect on my journey, I can't help but feel like I've been given a new lease on life. What started as a battle against Type 2 diabetes and weight challenges has turned into a transformative experience, reshaping not only my body but also my mind and spirit. The challenges I faced taught me resilience, the milestones I achieved gave me confidence, and the lessons I learned continue to guide me toward a healthier, happier future.

This transformation was never just about lowering blood sugar or shedding pounds. It was about reclaiming my life and becoming the best version of myself; physically, mentally, and emotionally. I now see my health not as a burden but as a source of strength and pride. Each day feels like a new opportunity to continue building on this foundation, living with purpose, and embracing the possibilities ahead.

## The Power of Letting Go

A significant turning point in my journey was cutting alcohol and sugar from my life. These changes were not easy, but they unlocked a level of clarity, stability, and joy I never thought possible. By removing these harmful substances, I discovered a new sense of balance that allowed me to focus on what truly matters: my health, my happiness, and the relationships that enrich my life.

Letting go of what no longer served me created space for new habits, new energy, and new perspectives. It was this clarity that empowered me to make better choices and sustain my progress. I've learned that treating my body with respect and care directly impacts my mental and emotional wellbeing.

## Celebrating the Journey

Every step forward, no matter how small, became a victory worth celebrating. From watching my blood sugar stabilize to walking longer distances without fatigue, each milestone reinforced my belief that I was capable of real change.

But the most meaningful victories weren't just physical; they were emotional. I gained the confidence to face my fears, the strength to overcome setbacks, and the self-love to forgive my imperfections. These moments of growth have become the true rewards of this journey; reminders that every effort, no matter how difficult, is part of something greater.

## Lessons to Carry Forward

As I close this chapter of my story, I want to leave you with the lessons that shaped my transformation:

**Small Steps, Big Changes:** Focus on consistency, not perfection. Even small changes can lead to profound results over time.

**Mindset Matters:** Embrace challenges as opportunities to grow. Your attitude will determine your success.

**Holistic Health:** True wellness includes the mind, body, and soul. Don't neglect any part of your wellbeing.

**Celebrate Progress:** Acknowledge every milestone, no matter how small; it's a testament to your hard work.

**Your Journey, Your Time:** Transformation takes time, but the rewards are worth every effort.

### A Message to You

If you're reading this, wondering if change is possible, let me assure you: it is. I started from a place of uncertainty and self-doubt, but with persistence and belief in myself, I turned my life around. If I can do it, so can you.

Take that first step, no matter how small. You don't need to have all the answers or wait for the perfect moment. Start where you are, with what you have, and trust that every effort you make is bringing you closer to a healthier, happier future.

## A New Chapter Awaits

This journey has been a profound transformation, but it's also a beginning. The changes I've made are not the end of the story but the foundation for a lifetime of growth and discovery.

As you finish this book, I hope you feel inspired to begin your own journey. Whether it's improving your health, finding balance, or reclaiming joy, the path is yours to take. And as you move forward, know that the challenges you face will only make your victories sweeter.

The next chapter of your life is waiting to be written. Turn the page, take that first step, and believe in the incredible power within you. Your transformation starts now.

13

# Chapter 13: Embracing a Healthier, Happier You

**C**onclusion:

As I reflect on my journey, one thing stands out above all: this was not just about reversing Type 2 diabetes or losing weight—it was about reclaiming my life. It was about making a promise to myself to prioritize my health, my happiness, and my future. If there's one message I want to leave you with, it's this: if I can do it, so can you.

The path to better health isn't always smooth. It's filled with challenges, setbacks, and moments of doubt. But each obstacle you face is an opportunity to learn, grow, and strengthen your resolve. You don't have to be perfect, and you don't need all the answers to start. The most important step is simply deciding that your health is worth the effort and committing to the journey—one day at a time.

Since my transformation, I've made it a priority to sustain my progress and stay proactive about my health. Regular check-ups with my doctor have become milestones of pride rather than dread. I'll never forget the last time I saw him—he was astonished by my results. My blood sugar levels were normal, my weight was stable, and I radiated energy and confidence. What's more, he began asking me for advice on how I'd achieved such remarkable changes.

Hearing my doctor say, "Yes, it can be done. "Well done," was a powerful moment. But the greatest reward wasn't just reversing diabetes—it was knowing that I'd regained control over my life. For the first time in years, I felt proud, empowered, and capable of achieving anything I set my mind to.

To you, my reader, I want to say this: don't wait for a diagnosis or a moment of crisis to take action. Your health is your greatest asset, and the time to protect and nurture it is now. Start where you are, with what you have, and focus on small, consistent changes. Every healthy choice you make—whether it's swapping out sugar, taking a brisk walk, or practicing mindfulness—brings you closer to the vibrant, fulfilling life you deserve.

This journey isn't just about your physical health; it's about discovering the strength and resilience that already exists within you. It's about redefining what's possible and unlocking the best version of yourself.

As you take your first steps, remember that progress, not perfection, is the goal. Celebrate your victories, no matter how small, and keep moving forward. The journey ahead may challenge you, but the rewards—a healthier body, a clearer mind, and a happier heart—are worth every effort.

So, let your transformation begin today. Believe in yourself, because you are capable, you are deserving, and you are enough. Your new chapter is waiting to be written, and it starts now.

Here's to your health, your happiness, and a brighter, more empowered future.

14

# Chapter 14: Final Thoughts and Support for Your Journey

Thank you for taking the time to read this guide. I hope the strategies and insights shared in these pages inspire and empower you on your journey to reversing Type 2 diabetes, improving your health, and achieving lasting transformation.

Remember, the path to success is not a sprint but a continuous journey of growth, consistency, and self-compassion. As someone who has walked this path, I understand the challenges and triumphs that come with making life-changing decisions. You have the strength and resilience to create a healthier, happier version of yourself. Embrace the process, celebrate your wins, big or small, and never stop striving for better.

**My Personal Support for You**

Your journey doesn't have to be a solitary one. I want to extend my support to you beyond the pages of this book. If you need personalized guidance or feel stuck along the way,

I'm here to help. I offer one-on-one consultations to provide tailored advice, answer your questions, and guide you through challenges. Whether it's managing blood sugar, maintaining motivation, building sustainable habits, addressing emotional well-being, or achieving weight loss goals, you can count on my experience to support you. Let's work together to create a plan that works for you.

To book a one-on-one session or reach out for support, contact me at: soweda@hotmail.com

Thanks for reading, and I wish you all the best!
*Shadi Oweda*

*[Images used in this document were sourced from Pexels and are free for commercial use. A special thank you to the photographers who have shared their work with the community.]*

# 15

# Recipes and Meal Plans

Sample Meal Plan for a Week

**Day 1:**

- **Breakfast**: Greek yogurt with mixed berries and a sprinkle of chia seeds.
- **Lunch**: Grilled chicken salad with mixed greens, cherry tomatoes, cucumbers, and a lemon vinaigrette.
- **Dinner**: Baked salmon with a side of quinoa and steamed broccoli.
- **Snacks**: A handful of almonds and an apple.

**Day 2:**

- **Breakfast**: Smoothie with spinach, banana, almond milk, and a scoop of protein powder.
- **Lunch**: Turkey and avocado wrap with whole-grain tor-

tilla.

- **Dinner**: Stir-fried tofu with mixed vegetables and brown rice.
- **Snacks**: Carrot sticks with hummus.

## Day 3:

- **Breakfast**: Oatmeal topped with fresh blueberries and a drizzle of honey.
- **Lunch**: Quinoa salad with black beans, corn, bell peppers, and a lime dressing.
- **Dinner**: Grilled shrimp with a side of roasted sweet potatoes and asparagus.
- **Snacks**: Greek yogurt with a handful of walnuts.

## Day 4:

- **Breakfast**: Scrambled eggs with spinach and tomatoes.
- **Lunch**: Lentil soup with a side of whole-grain bread.
- **Dinner**: Baked chicken breast with a side of cauliflower rice and green beans.
- **Snacks**: A pear and a handful of mixed nuts.

## Day 5:

- **Breakfast**: Smoothie bowl with mixed berries, banana, and a sprinkle of granola.
- **Lunch**: Chickpea salad with cucumbers, tomatoes, red onion, and feta cheese.
- **Dinner**: Grilled steak with a side of mashed cauliflower and sautéed spinach.

- **Snacks**: Celery sticks with almond butter.

## Day 6:

- **Breakfast**: Whole-grain toast with avocado and a poached egg.
- **Lunch**: Tuna salad with mixed greens, cherry tomatoes, and a balsamic vinaigrette.
- **Dinner**: Baked cod with a side of wild rice and steamed carrots.
- **Snacks**: A handful of grapes and a piece of dark chocolate.

## Day 7:

- **Breakfast**: Chia pudding with almond milk, topped with fresh strawberries.
- **Lunch**: Grilled vegetable wrap with whole-grain tortilla.
- **Dinner**: Turkey meatballs with a side of zucchini noodles and marinara sauce.
- **Snacks**: A small handful of trail mix.

## Recipes
### 1. Baked Salmon with Quinoa and Broccoli

- **Ingredients**:
- 2 salmon fillets
- 1 cup quinoa
- 2 cups broccoli florets
- 2 tbsp olive oil
- 1 lemon, sliced
- Salt and pepper to taste

- **Instructions**:

1. Preheat the oven to 375°F (190°C).
2. Place the salmon fillets on a baking sheet, drizzle with olive oil, and season with salt and pepper. Top with lemon slices.
3. Bake for 20-25 minutes until the salmon is cooked through.
4. Cook quinoa according to package instructions.
5. Steam broccoli until tender.
6. Serve the salmon with quinoa and broccoli on the side.

## 2. Greek Yogurt with Mixed Berries

- **Ingredients**:
- 1 cup Greek yogurt
- 1/2 cup mixed berries (blueberries, strawberries, raspberries)
- 1 tbsp chia seeds
- **Instructions**:

1. In a bowl, combine Greek yogurt and mixed berries.
2. Sprinkle chia seeds on top.
3. Enjoy as a healthy breakfast or snack.

# 16

# Exercise Routines

**B**eginner Exercise Routine
**Warm-Up (5-10 minutes)**

- Light jogging or brisk walking
- Arm circles
- Leg swings

**Strength Training (3 sets of each exercise)**

1. **Bodyweight Squats**: 15 reps
2. **Push-Ups**: 10 reps (modify by doing them on your knees if needed)
3. **Plank**: Hold for 30 seconds
4. **Lunges**: 10 reps per leg
5. **Dumbbell Rows**: 12 reps per arm (use a water bottle if you don't have dumbbells)

## Cardio (15-20 minutes)

- Brisk walking or light jogging
- Jumping jacks
- High knees

## Cool-Down (5-10 minutes)

- Stretching exercises for all major muscle groups
- Deep breathing exercises

## Intermediate Exercise Routine
## Warm-Up (5-10 minutes)

- Jump rope or brisk walking
- Dynamic stretches (leg swings, arm circles)

## Strength Training (3 sets of each exercise)

1. **Goblet Squats**: 15 reps (hold a dumbbell or kettlebell)
2. **Push-Ups**: 15 reps
3. **Plank with Shoulder Taps**: 20 taps (10 per shoulder)
4. **Walking Lunges**: 12 reps per leg
5. **Bent-Over Rows**: 15 reps per arm

## Cardio (20-25 minutes)

- Running or cycling
- Burpees
- Mountain climbers

## Cool-Down (5-10 minutes)

- Stretching exercises for all major muscle groups
- Deep breathing exercises

# 17

# Mindful Walking and Guided Visualization

**P**urpose: To practice mindfulness while engaging in physical activity.

**Instructions**:

1. Find a quiet place where you can walk without distractions.
2. Begin walking at a slow, steady pace.
3. Focus your attention on the sensation of your feet making contact with the ground.
4. Notice the movement of your legs, the rhythm of your steps, and the feeling of your body in motion.
5. If your mind starts to wander, gently bring your focus back to the act of walking.
6. Practice mindful walking for 10-15 minutes.

## Guided Visualization

**Purpose**: To reduce stress and promote relaxation through mental imagery.

**Instructions**:

1. Find a comfortable seated or lying position and close your eyes.
2. Take a few deep breaths to relax and center yourself.
3. Imagine a peaceful, calming place, such as a beach, forest, or meadow.
4. Visualize yourself in this place, taking in the sights, sounds, and smells.
5. Spend a few minutes exploring this place in your mind, noticing how it makes you feel.
6. When you are ready, take a few deep breaths and slowly open your eyes.

# 18

# Mindfulness and Meditation Exercises

**Mindful Breathing**

**Purpose**: To calm the mind and reduce stress by focusing on the breath.

**Instructions**:

1. Find a comfortable seated position with your back straight and your hands resting on your lap.
2. Close your eyes and take a deep breath in through your nose, filling your lungs completely.
3. Slowly exhale through your mouth, releasing any tension in your body.
4. Continue to breathe deeply and naturally, focusing your attention on the sensation of your breath entering and leaving your body.
5. If your mind starts to wander, gently bring your focus back to your breath.
6. Practice this mindful breathing for 5-10 minutes.

## Body Scan Meditation

**Purpose**: To increase body awareness and release physical tension.

**Instructions**:

1. Lie down on your back with your arms resting by your sides and your legs slightly apart.
2. Close your eyes and take a few deep breaths to relax.
3. Begin by focusing on your toes. Notice any sensations, tension, or discomfort.
4. Slowly move your attention up through your body, focusing on each part in turn: feet, ankles, calves, knees, thighs, hips, lower back, abdomen, chest, shoulders, arms, hands, neck, and head.
5. As you focus on each body part, take a deep breath in and imagine sending relaxation to that area. Exhale and release any tension.
6. Continue this body scan until you have covered your entire body.
7. Finish by taking a few deep breaths and slowly opening your eyes.

## Loving-Kindness Meditation

**Purpose**: To cultivate compassion and positive emotions towards oneself and others.

**Instructions**:

1. Find a comfortable seated position and close your eyes.
2. Take a few deep breaths to relax and center yourself.
3. Begin by silently repeating the following phrases to yourself: "May I be happy. May I be healthy. May I be safe. May I live with ease."
4. After a few minutes, shift your focus to someone you care about and repeat the phrases for them: "May you be happy. May you be healthy. May you be safe. May you live with ease."
5. Next, extend these wishes to someone you have neutral feelings towards, and then to someone you may have difficulty with.
6. Finally, extend these wishes to all beings everywhere: "May all beings be happy. May all beings be healthy. May all beings be safe. May all beings live with ease."
7. Take a few deep breaths and slowly open your eyes.

# 19

# Guided Visualization

**P****urpose**: To reduce stress and promote relaxation through mental imagery.
   **Instructions**:

1. Find a comfortable seated or lying position and close your eyes.
2. Take a few deep breaths to relax and center yourself.
3. Imagine a peaceful, calming place, such as a beach, forest, or meadow.
4. Visualize yourself in this place, taking in the sights, sounds, and smells.
5. Spend a few minutes exploring this place in your mind, noticing how it makes you feel.
6. When you are ready, take a few deep breaths and slowly open your eyes.

# 20

# Worksheets and Journals

## 1. Weekly Progress Tracker

**Worksheets and Journals**

**1. Weekly Progress Tracker**

| Week | Weight (kg) | Blood Sugar (mg/dL) | Exercise (minutes) | Notes |
| --- | --- | --- | --- | --- |
| 1 | | | | |
| 2 | | | | |
| 3 | | | | |
| 4 | | | | |

**Instructions**: Use this tracker to log your weight, blood sugar levels, and exercise duration each week. Add any notes about your progress, challenges, or achievements.

**2. Goal Setting Worksheet**

| Goal | Action Steps | Timeline | Progress |
|---|---|---|---|
| Example: Lose 5 kg | 1. Follow a balanced diet | 3 months | |
| | 2. Exercise 30 minutes daily | | |
| | 3. Track weight weekly | | |

**Instructions**: Write down your health goals, the action steps needed to achieve them, and the timeline for each goal. Track your progress regularly.

**3. Daily Journal Prompts**

- What healthy choices did I make today?
- How did I feel physically and emotionally today?
- What challenges did I face, and how did I overcome them?
- What am I grateful for today?
- What are my goals for tomorrow?

Use these to reflect on your daily experiences, track your progress, and stay motivated.

21

# Frequently Asked Questions (FAQs)

**1. What is Type 2 diabetes?**

Type 2 diabetes is a chronic condition that affects the way your body processes blood sugar (glucose). It occurs when your body becomes resistant to insulin or when the pancreas is unable to produce enough insulin to maintain normal glucose levels.

**2. Can Type 2 diabetes be reversed?**

Yes, Type 2 diabetes can be reversed through lifestyle changes such as a healthy diet, regular exercise, weight loss, and proper management of blood sugar levels. My doctor and I have personally proven this through my journey, and many others have successfully reversed their diabetes by adopting these changes.

## 3. What are the symptoms of Type 2 diabetes?

Common symptoms include increased thirst, frequent urination, fatigue, blurred vision, slow-healing sores, and unexplained weight loss. If you experience any of these symptoms, it's important to consult a healthcare professional.

## 4. How does diet impact Type 2 diabetes?

Diet plays a crucial role in managing Type 2 diabetes. Consuming a balanced diet with nutrient-dense foods, low glycemic index foods, and avoiding processed sugars and unhealthy fats can help regulate blood sugar levels and improve overall health.

## 5. What is intermittent fasting, and how does it help with diabetes?

Intermittent fasting (IF) is an eating pattern that cycles between periods of fasting and eating. It helps regulate blood sugar levels, promote fat loss, and improve metabolic health. IF can be an effective tool for managing and reversing Type 2 diabetes.

## 6. What types of foods should I include in my diet to manage diabetes?

Include foods rich in fiber, healthy fats, lean proteins, and low glycemic index carbohydrates. Examples include leafy green vegetables, nuts, berries, whole grains, lean meats, and healthy fats like olive oil and avocado.

## 7. How important is exercise in managing Type 2 diabetes?

Exercise is essential for managing Type 2 diabetes. Regular physical activity helps improve insulin sensitivity, lower blood sugar levels, and promote weight loss. Activities like walking, jogging, resistance training, and yoga can be beneficial.

## 8. How can I stay motivated to maintain a healthy lifestyle?

Staying motivated can be challenging, but setting realistic goals, tracking your progress, celebrating milestones, and seeking support from family, friends, or online communities can help. Remember to focus on the long-term benefits of a healthier lifestyle.

## 9. What role does sleep play in managing diabetes?

Quality sleep is crucial for regulating insulin resistance, metabolism, and emotional health. Poor sleep can disrupt these processes, leading to higher blood sugar levels and increased cravings. Prioritizing restorative sleep can significantly improve diabetes management.

## 10. How can mindfulness and stress management help with diabetes?

Mindfulness and stress management techniques, such as meditation, deep breathing, and yoga, can help reduce stress and anxiety, which can negatively impact blood sugar levels. Incorporating these practices into your routine can support overall health and diabetes management.

## 11. What should I do if I experience setbacks in my health journey?

Setbacks are a natural part of any health journey. It's important to stay positive, learn from the experience, and make necessary adjustments to your diet, exercise, or lifestyle. Seek support from healthcare professionals, family, or support groups to stay on track.

## 12. How can I track my progress in managing Type 2 diabetes?

Use tools like blood sugar monitoring apps, weight tracking apps, and fitness trackers to monitor your progress. Regularly logging your readings and analyzing trends can help you make informed adjustments to your lifestyle and stay motivated.

# 22

# Glossary of Terms

**1. Blood Glucose**: The main sugar found in the blood and the body's primary source of energy. Also known as blood sugar.

**2. Insulin**: A hormone produced by the pancreas that helps regulate blood glucose levels by facilitating the uptake of glucose into cells.

**3. Glycemic Index (GI)**: A measure of how quickly a food causes blood glucose levels to rise. Foods with a low GI are digested and absorbed more slowly, leading to a gradual rise in blood sugar.

**4. HbA1c**: A blood test that measures the average blood glucose levels over the past 2-3 months. It is used to diagnose and monitor diabetes.

**5. Intermittent Fasting (IF)**: An eating pattern that cycles between periods of fasting and eating. Common methods include the 16:8 method, where you fast for 16 hours and eat during an 8-hour window.

**6. Insulin Resistance**: A condition in which the body's cells become less responsive to insulin, leading to higher blood glucose levels.

**7. Metabolism**: The chemical processes that occur within the body to maintain life, including the conversion of food into energy.

**8. Mindfulness**: The practice of being present and fully engaged in the current moment, without judgment.

**9. Type 2 Diabetes**: A chronic condition characterized by high blood glucose levels due to insulin resistance or insufficient insulin production.

**10. Nutrient-Dense Foods**: Foods that are high in nutrients but relatively low in calories. Examples include vegetables, fruits, lean proteins, and whole grains.

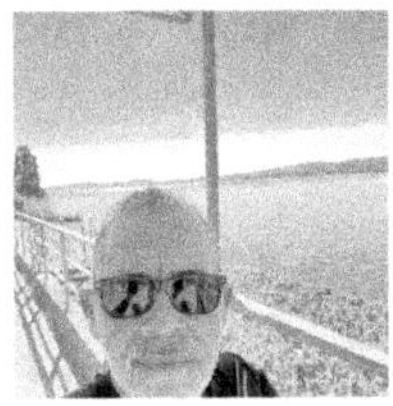

# About the Author

**Shadi Oweda** is a seasoned ICT consultant, productivity expert, online instructor, and e-commerce consultant with over 30 years of experience.  After being diagnosed with Type 2 diabetes, Shadi embarked on a transformative journey to reclaim his health. Through determination, self-research, and a commitment to change, he successfully reversed his condition and achieved lasting weight loss.  Shadi is now dedicated to sharing his knowledge and practical solutions to help others break free from the constraints of diabetes and achieve sustainable, long-term health and wellness.

# Also by Shadi Oweda

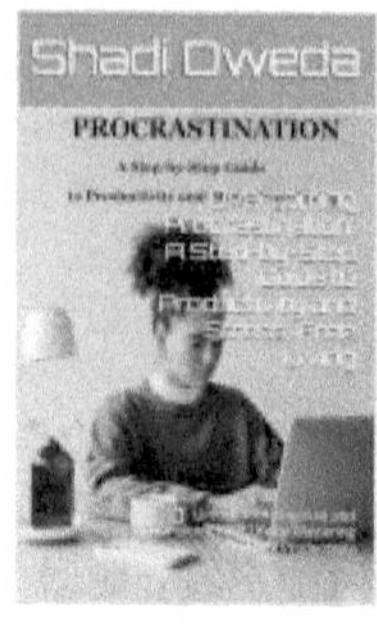

**Overcoming Procrastination A Step-by-Step Guide to Productivity and Stress-Free Living**
**Overcoming Procrastination: A Step-by-Step Guide to Productivity and Stress-Free Living**

Are you tired of constantly putting things off and feeling overwhelmed by your to-do list? In "Overcoming Procrastination," Shadi Oweda shares practical strategies and actionable steps to help you break free from the cycle of procrastination. This comprehensive guide will empower you to boost your productivity, reduce stress, and achieve your goals with confidence. Discover the secrets to a more organized, efficient, and fulfilling life. Start your journey to productivity and stress-free living today!